BODY-CENTERED PSYCHOTHERAPY
The Hakomi Method

The Integrated Use of
Mindfulness, Nonviolence and the Body

RON KURTZ

LIFERHYTHM

Lines from:
Faith and Violence: Christian Teaching and Christian Practice by Thomas Merton. Copyright © 1968 by University of Notre Dame Press. Used by permission of the publisher.
Webster's II New Riverside University Dictionary. Copyright © 1988 by Houghton Mifflin Co. Adapted and reprinted by permission from Webster's II New Riverside University Dictionary.
Evolution: The Grand Synthesis by Ervin Laszlo. Copyright © 1987. Reprinted by arrangement with Shambhala Publications, Inc., 300 Mass. Ave., Boston, MA 02115.
Awakening the Heart by John Welwood. Copyright © 1983. Reprinted by arrangement with Shambhala Publications, Inc., 300 Mass Ave., Boston, MA 02115.
The Tree of Knowledge: The Biological Roots of Human Understanding by Humberto R. Maturana and Francisco J. Varela. Copyright © 1987. Reprinted by arrangement with Shambhala Publications, Inc., 300 Mass. Ave., Boston, MA 02115.
Tao Te Ching by Lao Tsu. Copyright © 1972 by Gia-Fu Feng and Jane English, Translators. Reprinted by Permission of Alfred A. Knopf, Inc.
Godel, Escher, Bach, An Eternal Golden Braid by Douglas R. Hofstadter. Copyright © 1979 by Basic Books, Inc. Reprinted by permission of Basic Books, Inc., Publishers.
The Body Electric by Robert Becker and Gary Selden. Copyright © 1985 by Dr. Robert Becker and Gary Selden. Reprinted by permission of William Morrow & Co., Inc.
Eye to Eye by Ken Wilbur. Copyright © 1983. Reprinted by arrangement with Sobel Weber Associates, Inc.
A Talk by Ilya Prigogine, reprinted with permission from Ilya Prigogine.
"Believing is Seeing—Not the Reverse" by Edward T. Clark, in *Quest Magazine*, Autumn, 1988. Reprinted by Permission from Quest Magazine.
On Growth and Form by D'Arcy Thompson. Copyright © 1952. Reprinted by permission from Cambridge University Press.
The Miracle of Mindfulness by Nhat Hanh. Copyright © 1976. Reprinted by permission from Beacon Press, Publisher.
Three Plays by Ugo Betti. Copyright © 1958. From "The Burnt Flower Bed", reprinted by permission from Grove Press.
The Psychobiology of Mind-Body Healing by Ernest Rossi. Copyright © 1986. Reprinted with permission from W.W. Norton & Co.
The Self-Organizing Universe by Erich Jantsch. Copyright © 1986. Reprinted with permission from Pergamon Press PLC.
Great and Small by Chuang Tzu, taken from *When the Shoe Fits* by Bhagwan Shree Rajneesh. Copyright © 1976. Reprinted by permission from Chidvilas Inc.
Ever Since Darwin by Stephen Jay Gould. Copyright © 1977. Reprinted by permission of W.W. Norton & Co., Inc.
Planet Medicine by Richard Grossinger. Copyright © 1985. Reprinted by permission from the author and North Atlantic Books, Berkeley, California.
The Dharma That Illuminates All Being by Kalu Rinpoche. Copyright © 1986. Reprinted by permission of State University of New York Press.
Creative Use of Emotion by Swami Rama and Swami Ajaya. Copyright © 1976. Reprinted by permission from the Himalayan International Institute.
The Potent Self by Moshe Feldenkrais. Copyright © 1985. Reprinted by permission of Harper & Row, Publishers, Inc. (world rights except Israel)
Infinite in All Directions by Freeman Dyson. Copyright © 1988 by Freeman Dyson. Reprinted by permission of Harper & Row, Publishers, Inc. (world rights).
"Good, Wild, Sacred", by Gary Snyder, printed in *Meeting the Expectations of the Land*, Copyright © 1984 by Wes Jackson, editor. Published by North Point Press and reprinted by permission.
The Power of Mindfulness by Nyanaponika Thera. Copyright © 1972 by Buddhist Publication Society, Kandy, Shri Lanka.
"Directive", a poem by Robert Frost,1947, 1969 by Holt, Rinehart and Winston. Copyright © 1975 by Lesley Frost Ballantine. Reprinted from *The Poetry of Robert Frost* edited by Edward Connery Lathem, by permission of Henry Holt & Co., Inc.
The Reenchantment of the World by Morris Berman. Copyright © 1983. Reprinted by permission of Cornell University Press.
The Gestalt Approach and Eyewitness Therapy by Fritz Perls. © 1979. Reprinted by permission of Science and Behavior Books.
Mind and Nature by Gregory Bateson. Copyright © 1979. Reprinted by permission of E.P. Dutton.
The Origin of Consciousness in the Breakdown of the Bicameral Mind by Julian Jaynes. Copyright © 1977. Reprinted by permission of Houghton Mifflin Co.

Library of Congress Cataloging-in-Publication Data
Kurtz, Ron
    Body-centered psychotherapy: the Hakomi method.
    Includes bibliographies.
    1. Mind and body therapies. I Title
[DNLM: 1. Psychotherapy—methods. WM 420 K965b]
RC489.M53K88 1990 615.8'51 89-13250
ISBN 0-940795-03-5 Paperback edition   ISBN 0-940795-18-3 Hardcover edition

Type Design: William Wise
Cover Design: Mark Gatter and Siegmar Gerken
Photographs on p. 197 and p. 212 by Morgan Alexander

Dedication

Terry and Lily,
Swami Rama and Meher Baba:
teachers of love.

TABLE OF CONTENTS

SECTION TWO: PROCESS

Acknowledgments

I would like to offer my appreciation to all those who helped bring this book into being, but due to the unbroken wholeness of the natural world, I can only mention a very few. William Wise for his tremendous efforts around format and layout. Cathy Black, Meg Cole, Allan Davidson, Lucky Del Prince, Jack Eagleson, Jon Eisman, Dan Henderson, and Jim Schulman for their ideas, editing and constant support. Tim Flatt for his layout suggestions. For all the years we've learned and taught together, and for all the love that went with it, Cedar Barstow, Dyrian Benz, Lucky Del Prince, Jon Eisman, Richy Heckler, Morgan Holford, Greg Johanson, Amina Knowlan, Roland Kopp, Pat Ogden, Devi Records, Rainer Scheunemann, Jim Schulman, Martin Schulmeister and Halko Weiss. Siegmar Gerken, my ever energetic publisher, Dixie Shipp and Sharon Bolles, who together chased down and got permission for all the quotes. To my students, I am grateful. Finally, to my wife, Terry Toth, without whom it just wouldn't have been worth it.

The Word Hakomi

In the summer of 1980, nineteen of us gathered to study this work and to start an institute. We also tried to find a name. We tried brainstorming and only got silly each time. Finally, David Winters had a dream in which I handed him a piece of paper with the words "Hakomi Therapy" on it. The word was meaningless then to all of us, though David thought it might be an Amerindian word. David went home, an eight-hour trip, and looked the word up in some reference books he had back there. He discovered it was a Hopi Indian word (sometimes spelled hakimi) with two related meanings. Its current usage is "who are you." It's archaic meaning is "how do you stand in relation to these many realms." That suited us to a tee, so we took it. Since, I have heard of its meanings and possible meanings in Chinese (universal, reverent laughter) and Hebrew (this is my... place, existence, becoming, setting up). In 1981, I made a trip to southern Colorado to find Grandfather David of the Hopi Nations, seeking his counsel on David's dream and our institute's use of a Hopi word. I missed him by a few hours. I never made another opportunity, but with the publication of this book, I feel I must try again.

Preface

The unfolding and growth of consciousness is the central process of psychology and, in one viewpoint, of every human life, all history and the evolution of the cosmos. From the sea of atoms, an incomprehensibly large number of living beings have emerged. In their capacity to create and recreate there is a knowing, an awareness of self, binding order from the flow of chance and mischance. With each unfolding of the drama, cosmic or personal, consciousness grows - as central player, as the ground of being, whether in the few brief hours of psychotherapy, or in any single lifetime rich with experiences, or set against the vast reaches of time and space upon which the galaxies parade.

Psychotherapy brings a useful harmony to the functions of the mind, the body and the exigencies of the outer world. In the sweep and richness of its language, the precision and delicacy of its techniques, its caring, its power to inform and in the heart wrenching beauty of its finest moments, it is both high art and ancient science. To know it and to live it has been a great gift that God has given me. I would share that gift with all the world.

This book represents my efforts over the last decade to make the work I do teachable. Throughout, I am trying to make clear to myself as much as to the reader, each aspect I've discovered - principles, guidelines, relationship, patterns, techniques, method - the entire structure of the work as I now know it. I keep growing, so this is only a pause to collect the thinking of the last ten years. It is not complete. Already I am looking beyond, to the worlds of order and chaos, and the principles of heuristics put forth by Emanuel Peterfreund.

I have tried to make conscious what was at first, intuitive and only vaguely felt. Not to take the art out of it, but to help others to be artful with it.

This book was completed in May of 1989, in the countryside near Ashland, Oregon.

Ron Kurtz

SECTION ONE

THE CONTEXT

So, when the shoe fits
the foot is forgotten

when the belt fits
the belly is forgotten

when the heart is right
"for" and "against" are forgotten.

Chuang Tzu

INTRODUCTION
PART 1:

THE PRINCIPLES AND THE METHOD OF EVOKED EXPERIENCES

Our ordinary consciousness is not "natural," but an acquired product. This has given us both many useful skills and many insane sources of useless suffering.

– Charles Tart, Waking Up

Evocation: creation anew by way of imagination or memory.

– Webster's II New Riverside Dictionary

You can't do what you want till you know what you're doing.

– Moshe Feldenkrais, A favorite saying

Fifty thousand years ago it must have been easy to be an absolutist. You weren't likely to run into anyone who looked, spoke, dressed or thought very different from you or anyone else you knew. Now, the easiest thing in the world is to find someone or something different. And the differences are staggering. Endless lines of near naked Africans are starving in their dry land just a two-hour flight from the docked yachts of Monaco. At home in Toledo or Tashkent, we watch it all on TV.

This closeness is giving our present day absolutists a hard time. (And as usual, they are giving everybody else a hard time.) After thousands of centuries of slow, relatively isolated development, we are experiencing a forced, potentially explosive fusion of deeply ingrained, conflicting ideas, customs, laws and languages. From a global perspective, we live in tension and diversity everywhere. That tension is killing millions and exhausting the world's resources. It is a time for change. It is a time for relativists, for generalists, for holists, for people who love diversity, a time to find beauty in the whole and meanings we can all agree on.

There are such people in almost every field: philosophy, science, medicine, theology. We are in the middle of the revolution that they are making. They are offering us something new — not our usual way of knowing, being and doing. It is a vision coming into focus, a "second language" we are still learning. The new paradigm does not deny the past. On the contrary, it's most significant contribution will be to integrate past and present and to make common sense of the great diversity of our inherited wisdom. It is a comprehensive "spiritual/philosophic/ scientific system." It is incomplete and only just beginning to affect us. Wherever we're going, we surely are not yet there. Still, the voyage has begun and the direction is clear enough.

The **Hakomi Method of Body/Mind Therapy** is grounded in a set of principles that reflect this revolution or what is often called the shifting paradigm. The work is just one inspired expression of these principles. Our methods and techniques, the relationships we develop with our clients and each other, are all expressions of the principles, scaled down to meet each task and moment of the work. They are about holism, unity and a participatory universe; about relationship; about the nature of living beings and their differences from the material, mechanical realm. They are about the reality of consciousness and its place in therapy. They are about the effectiveness of nonviolence. They are the "dharma" of Hakomi, its source of wisdom, clarity and power. These principles are the heart of the work and a refuge for therapists lost.

My first concern as a teacher of Hakomi is that my students understand and work within the principles. It is this that makes their work clean and effective. I invite and encourage them to make the principles a consistent part of who they are and how they work, to let the principles inform each aspect of the their process: learning, personal development and therapeutic practice. The principles are a whole world, having as much to do with becoming full human beings as with doing therapy; as much about therapy as about the universe or how to cook a small fish or meet another human soul.

Hakomi also has some ideas about people. People are living beings, different in fundamental ways from the machines. We are self-organizing. We are systems that self-create and self-maintain. We heal. Machines don't do that. So, we look at people as self-organizing systems, organized psychologically around core memories, beliefs and images. This core material is at the very heart of what we have made of our lives. It creates and maintains our images of self and of our culturally acquired world. It directs our perceptions and actions. Core material expresses itself through all the habits and attitudes which make us individuals. Our feelings, actions and perceptions are continuously influenced by core material around major themes: safety and belonging; support, love and appreciation; freedom and responsibility; openness and honesty; control, power, sexuality, membership, and the social and cultural rules. These themes are the daily grist of therapeutic work.

Hakomi is a method for helping people change their way of being in the world through working with core material and changing core beliefs. It is a transformational method and it follows a general outline: First, we work to build a relationship which maximizes safety and the cooperation of the unconscious. With that relationship, we help the client focus on and study how he or she organizes experience. Most behavior is habit, automatically organized by core material. Thus, when we study the organization of experience, we are studying the influence of this core material. It is usually a simple step from that to direct contact with core feelings, beliefs and memories.

To study the organization of experience, we establish and use a state of consciousness called *mindfulness*. Many books have been written on mindfulness; it is part of every transpersonal tradition we know about. It is a distinct state of consciousness, characterized by relaxed volition, a surrender to and acceptance of the happenings of the moment, a gentle, sustained focus of attention inward, a heightened sensitivity and the ability to observe and name the contents of consciousness. It is self-reflective. It is doubtful that any other species, with the possible exception of whales, dolphins and the great apes, are even capable of it. Though we humans are capable, we don't seem to be doing it all that much. When we do, we are able to gather information about ourselves with relative ease. In psychotherapy, nothing is more useful than mindfulness.

In mindfulness, therapist and client together create and use evoked experiences. When the client indicates that he or she is ready, the therapist introduces an "external influence" into this quiet, self-observing state. The influence can be a statement about a key theme, an image, a touch, or a sound. It can even be suggestion that the client say something or do something, such as a clear, slow movement. As long as the client is able to allow and notice his or her reactions, the method works.

For example, the client could be slowly raising an arm upward in a real or imagined context of reaching out to someone, all the while studying the experience thus created. Perhaps, at some point in the arm's travel, the client notices fear. Casually and quickly raising the arm, especially if it is part of doing something like getting a jar down off the shelf, won't evoke that fear. It is mindfulness — the slowness of the action, the self-observing and the focus on experience (rather than the contents of the jar or thoughts about the recipe) that does the job. The fear most likely relates to memories and beliefs about reaching out to others. Following the evocation of the fear (or whatever experience is evoked), a transition to processing takes place, if the client is ready.

Processing is state-specific, because core material, especially core organizing memories, are state-specific. There are three different states we work with: mindfulness; strong emotions; and a state in which a child-like consciousness appears. We use different methods with each.

The basic method is: create a relationship which allows the client to establish mindfulness, evoke experiences in that mindful state, and process the experiences evoked. All else that we do is done in support of this primary process. In order to evoke, we establish mindfulness. Once evoked, we process the experiences. In processing, we use the experiences evoked to help the client understand and change. All our methods and techniques conspire to bring this simple sequence to fruition. We create a safe, healing relationship in order to enable mindfulness. We use mindfulness to enhance sensitivity. We want sensitivity in order to go deep, to evoke experiences reflecting core emotional attitudes and beliefs. Our methods are simple in this light; they are all about creating and using evoked experiences to work with core material.

These methods are appropriate and effective in all kinds of therapeutic situations, such as work with couples, families, movement and bodywork. As a method, it is general and wide ranging, but it finds its full potential in personal and transpersonal growth. It is most useful when we commit to moving beyond our personal limits -- beyond the "insane sources of useless suffering" — to the full expression of who we are and what is possible.

Such growth is difficult. Core material goes deep; organizing beliefs are held firmly and defended strongly. Any attempt to force change is more than likely to fail. You cannot talk people out of long and deeply held conceptions about life and themselves. Organizing beliefs determine how we function. Like personal myths, they energize and give direction to behavior. They protect us against loss and pain. Such protection is not easily surrendered. You may give a client logical reasons to believe he is safe or lovable or whatever. You may tell him that no one is after him and that it is foolish to believe otherwise. The facts themselves may be obvious, even to him. And, if you're gentle enough and compassionate enough to avoid an atmosphere of confrontation, the client may even agree with you. Yet even as he does, he is still sweating; his teeth are still chattering; he still refuses to leave his house. Intellectually, the client may recognize that you are right. He may even say, "Yes. Of course. You're right. There really is nothing to be afraid of." But his physiology and his behavior say all too clearly, "There is!. There is!" Core material is not accessible through the intellect. But it is through mindfulness and evocation. For that reason, we work in non-ordinary states of consciousness.

Each of us organizes to meet the world in our own way. We give unique, personal meaning to what we receive from the world. Like wind chimes in the breeze, the sounds evoked tell more about the instrument than the wind. Evoked experiences are more about ourselves than the conditions that evoke them. In any situation, any two of us may have completely different, even opposite, experiences. Experience mirrors internal organization. It reflects memories and beliefs and those images of self and world which organize all experience. With mindful evocation we move close. Just a step or two, a question, a gesture, staying a little longer with the experience, and we are at the core.

People hardly ever treat evoked experiences as speculative. They immediately accept such experiences as real and significant. Experience is not easily doubted. Theories may be doubted, but not experiences. If the therapy process is kept on track, therapist and client do not talk about what might be true or how it all may have started. Both are engaged in what is happening right now. Core material is constantly and actively shaping present experience. It is operative and tangible. The special work of therapy makes it available to consciousness where, from a greater sense of self, it can be explored, understood, challenged and revised.

PART 2:

CHANGE WITHOUT FORCE

*... the kind of activity which dominates the instability phase
introduces a directedness, a vector which already indicates
in which direction the new structure may be expected.*

– Erich Jantsch, The Self-Organizing Universe

... every act of knowing brings forth a world.

– H. Maturana and F. Varela, The Tree of Knowledge

*True love is no game of the faint-hearted and the weak. It
is born of strength and understanding.*

– Meher Baba, on a poster

Hakomi is a non-violent psychotherapy. It is a way to help people change that allows for the wisdom and healing power in each of us. To work nonviolently, we must drop notions about making clients change and, along with that, any tendency to take credit for their successes. That doesn't mean we have to be passive; nonviolence is not inaction. We can work without using force or the ideas and methods of a paradigm of force. The question then is: If we don't use force, what do we use? How do we participate in the process of change without imposing our own agendas, without seeing ourselves as heroes — even in the most subtle way? Here's my thinking about that.

More than just growth, we want to participate in the client's evolution, in his or her natural movement toward full human-beingness. Carl Jung once remarked that patients don't get cured, they simply move on. Our job as therapists is to help them do that, to move on, to let go of whatever it is that blocks their way. We are there to help them: first, as they reach out toward what they might achieve, then as they struggle and work for their full humanity and finally, when they come to it. This is very special work. In this process, violence is not only useless, it is inevitably harmful.

In all evolution, there is pressure. The flow of water offers us a simple model. If you turn a water spigot slowly, the water at first comes out in a smooth, clear stream. The amount of water moving through is not enough to create turbulence. As the pressure increases, the water can no longer get through in this simple way. The water must do something to accommodate. It does; it braids. This braiding allows more water to flow through the space provided. Braiding is a more complex dynamic structure than the simple, clear flow we started with. In system theory terms, the flow has escaped to a higher order of complexity. It has evolved.

In the evolution of living beings there is a readiness, a waiting, as a seed waits for the length of days. The moisture and the warmth become signals, a calling forth and a promise to provide. "Come," it says, "be what you can be. Now. I am here. Come." Seeds know the endless cycle of the seasons, seed to sprout, plant, flower, seed. Evolving, stage after stage, knowing each call, ready for each. The cycle is the fullness.

Evolution is an act of courage. The seed has only the promise, only the signal. It is an act of faith, a leap into uncertainty. The seedling must emerge from its strong, protective sheath and venture forth. It is a time of vulnerability and danger. If conditions change, the seed is lost. I would agree — growth and change seem inevitable. It seems we must. Still, some people don't. And for those who do, it is choosing life, and that takes courage... especially when the pain of having failed before is part of who you are.

Character is growth delayed. Something was ready, but conditions weren't right. The right signals weren't there. The confidence, the sense of fullness never came or was cut off before it had a chance. Support was missing. The promise was betrayed. Now, years later, the client comes for therapy. Perhaps the readiness is back. Or it is close, prefigured in some way, but not yet conscious. Perhaps the promise is reborn, a new calling forth, the ripeness come round again.

So, that's the setting: readiness, remembered pain, a chance to grow. How do we participate in that, without violence, without force, with only our caring and wisdom and the truth of who we are as people? We do it by providing warmth and understanding, by creating a proper setting for a re-emergence of courage and vulnerability. We do it by recognizing those aspects of the client that are ripe for growth, encouraging and supporting that ripening. And finally, we do it by grace and magic and the simple authority of bearing witness and knowing the true names of things.

If we are not going to use force, we must use our ability to wait for the right moment, to recognize what is growing here and what is ready for expression. In therapy, this is the highest skill: to know each moment for what it can be. At the simplest level, it is noticing, perhaps a slight change in the tone of voice, a moistening of the eyes and naming that. "Some sadness, huh?" That knowing and naming brings the client to a place where he or she can open to the movement of tears and emotion and self-recognition that, left unmentioned, would have been held back. Something important and painful would have sunk back into the shadows, unspoken and unseen. To gently name what is real here and now, to speak out simply, without arguing or proving, that is not force. It is a wise and graceful use of the energies of the moment. It calls forth what is true in the client. And that is magic—the calling forth by naming. It has the authority of truth, truth spoken cleanly, with no other motive than to be present and bear witness.

On many levels, this presence and naming is our participation. We can name what is true for us, even to the point of recognizing a moment where we do not feel adequate to the task at hand. Even that will help the ripening. Beyond naming the experience of this moment, we can acknowledge the experience of a whole lifetime. Or we can "jump out of the system" and name what's been going on between ourselves and the client in a particular session or over a whole series of sessions. The truth, spoken with compassion, invites reply and welcomes memory and feeling. Each true naming infuses its particular moment with possibilities. "Every act of knowing brings forth a world."

Some part of the client already knows this truth, knows the holding back and the longing to move on. Because we have witnessed and spoken that truth, from a loving place, the client's way of dealing with it can be transformed. The client may have been dealing with this truth by hiding it from everyone, including himself. In therapy, it becomes evolution. Energies once invested in limiting the self are set free to animate the new.

Naming is just one influence of our gentle way. The love we bring, the compassion and respect we offer, these too are the proper setting for the client's unfolding. When we ask clients to be mindful, we are asking for vulnerability, for an openness to whatever will emerge. This may be their first dropping of the protective sheath. Mindfulness is both passive and open, a deeper sensitivity and a small act of courage in its own right. To help establish mindfulness, we have to be safe, supportive and loving. We must be a brother or a sister soul, nurturing and helping to make way for greater acts of courage yet to come. For beyond this vulnerability of mindfulness, there is the vulnerability of the child. This child is hurting and discouraged, memories full of loss and defeat, stung with isolation and numbing conflict. When we name these things, we name them with a heart that knows them, that knows their weight and knows what yet may come.

When the client finds wisdom and caring in a therapist, the unconscious responds. The child inside wants terribly to understand, wants to know what is real and what to do, to make sense of pain. In those moments, deep change is possible. There is an intensity, a still expectancy. In those moments, the needs and questions and possibilities of the child re-emerge. Growth is rekindled. A lost piece of the self is found and returned to its rightful place. After a long, silent journey, a member of the family has come home. The reward for all this difficult and painful work is simply knowing, from a place deep within, how one has come to this moment... and how one will move on.

None of this is force. Or it is force of a different kind, a part of life's elemental interconnectedness, life's constant birthing, its sweetness, its truth and overflowing love, stronger than worlds and the passing of time.

1

THE ORGANIZATION OF EXPERIENCE

When the only tool you have is a hammer, every problem looks like a nail.

- Abraham Maslow

...one of the conclusions that directs the cutting edge research in quantum physics is that the way that we perceive the universe to be — that is, the way we measure, describe and explain it — is, in some fundamentally significant way, a reflection of our Minds.

- Edward T. Clark, Jr.
Believing Is Seeing - Not the Reverse

P sychotherapy has been called, "the talking cure." Over the past few decades, the nature of that talking has changed dramatically. Psycho-therapy used to be talking about — about feelings, about relationships, the past, or anything else the client wanted to talk about. In that way it was a lot like any other kind of talking. It was conversational. Talking like that, talking about oneself and one's experience is often helpful. Sharing painful memories helps. But it also can be a long, slow, not so helpful process. It doesn't always touch deep issues. It doesn't focus directly on experiences in the present. Focusing on present experience, especially on emotional expression, came later. It came with Reichian Therapy, Psychodrama, Gestalt, encounter groups and all that followed. At that point, much of psychotherapy moved from merely talking about experiences to actually having them. Clients went from talking to working. And the work involved getting back into our bodies, our senses, below our minds, away from theories, away from talk/talk/talk and into experiences.

A lot of it happened in the sixties and was part of the great leap into being alive that was the crux of the sixties. Being alive basically meant having experiences. At Esalen Institute the battle cry was, do it! Don't just talk about it. Do it! Don't tell me about your anger. Show it to me! Yell and bang and make some noise! Into it! Live it! Enough of this energy draining, deadening talk. Get some aliveness into it! Get your energy going! Do it! As a result, things got done, adventurous things, like going to India, buying buses, being on the road, trying drugs, new sexual patterns and all the rest. It was all too ardent and full of life to call it simply, experimental. It was that, yes, but it had the feel and flavor of high adventure. When Perls told people to exaggerate their movements or voices, he was working to deepen the experience, to get to feelings, to get to a live experience and away from talk. The method was to interrupt any attempt to "head trip." And it worked. It gave the world wonderful new ways to do psychotherapy.

The shift towards experience was also a shift towards the present, where experience is. In encounter, one of the rules was: talk only about what is going on here and now, at this time, in this room. Stay in the present. In Gestalt Therapy the task was, stay in the here and now. (Just as the task in psychoanalysis was, free associate.) It added up to this: get into your experience, stay in it, exaggerate it and learn from it! And don't expect me to do any of that for you. This was a definite break with the old model.

In the 80's, the therapies at the cutting edge, like Feldenkrais and NLP, took the shift one step further. These therapies deal not only with experience but, more importantly, they deal with the organization of experience. In meditation, for example, we study what follows what in the flow of mental life, how the mind puts experiences together. In these new ways of the working, we're still having experiences, but we're not *just* having them. We're also studying how experiences are organized. We're studying the systems that put experience itself together. The goal of this new therapy is to contact and understand the events which create and maintain the flow of experience itself. We do it in order to transform the way we organize all experiences. This therapy is transformational.

In a study of master therapists, like Milton Erickson, Virginia Satir and others, it turned out that they held certain assumptions in common. The most surprising, to me, of these was the assumption that there is no real problem. The client may feel that there is a problem, but the master therapist "knows" there isn't. Why is that? Because: if it's a lovely day and there's nothing immediate to handle, and one person is enjoying that while at the same time someone else is having a terrible time, the difference isn't in the day, it is in what each of them is making out of it. It is the way each is organizing that beautiful day into their separate experiences. It is in the organization of experience. The problem isn't real. As Moshe Feldenkrais was so fond of telling us, "You can't do what you want, till you know what you're doing." When you know how you are organizing your experience, you become free to organize it in new ways. When you change not just what you experience, but how you experience, you have transcended, you have become a different self. You have transcended the habits and beliefs you were stuck in and controlled by. You now have new options. You do things and feel things in new ways. You have changed at the level of character. Your personal paradigm has shifted. This is how psychotherapy has changed. In Hakomi, we don't just talk about experiences. We don't just have experiences. Rather, we study how each of us organizes his or her experience.

Two entirely different processes determine what each of us experiences. One is what is actually happening around us and the second, the habits that convert these events into information, up the levels of the nervous system into progressively more complex, organized gestalts, and finally into consciousness. The lower, sensory levels are not usually problematic for psychotherapy. It is at the levels of meaning and feeling that the conversion of events into experience becomes highly individual, creative, distinctly human and sometimes unnecessarily painful and limiting.

In Hakomi, we help our clients study how they create meaning and feeling out of events, that is, how they organize their experiences. Whole classes of experiences are organized around key issues like safety or being loved. To study these, we first focus on a particular present experience, like a muscle tension pattern, a feeling or an image. This experience serves as a current example of experience being organized and is an access route to the core material behind it.

The logic of this process is simple. But, as simple as it is, it requires skills that run counter to everyday habits, especially the habits of ordinary conversation.

If you let the client take all the time he or she wants to describe what happened last week or last year, and if you stay very long with this talking about the past, you may end up listening, sympathetically perhaps, or offering commentary, but you'll have a very hard time doing anything about the things you are hearing. Talking in a conversational manner about feelings and events greatly limits what interventions are possible. If the client is talking about something that felt terrible yesterday or ten years ago, what can be done about that now? The therapeutic benefits are limited. Okay, it just feels good to talk to someone who knows how to listen with caring and intelligence. A sympathetic ear may help one to feel better for a while. The client may feel understood. It may help the client to feel the events again, to express buried emotions and to unburden herself or himself or to understand things better. Finally the client may have felt the same feelings in the past as he or she is feeling in the present experience and may gather insights from that about how past events influence what he or she does in the present. All that is helpful, but limited. The effects gradually filter down into the unconscious. But, when the therapy process takes place within ordinary conversation and ordinary consciousness, it is not nearly as effective as it could be. Therapy can be much more rapid and powerful.

Therapy isn't conversation. We need to distinguish between conversation and the work that clients and therapists do when the task is studying the organization of experience. We need a clear description of that task. Without one, therapist and client get stuck in the rituals of polite conversation. Because we seem to be just talking, we assume without thinking about it, that we must follow the rules and format of ordinary conversation. That's wrong and it's trouble. For this ridiculously simple reason: the rules of polite conversation are designed to expedite the flow of information between people, not within people. Eye movements, pauses, head turns and habits all control who speaks when and how much. The polite listener does not interrupt the speaker to ask for some experiment. The polite listener doesn't take charge of the conversation and tell the other what to say or do, telling the other to focus on some feeling or to focus awareness in one place or another. Yet this is exactly what therapists must do. We must help clients turn inward and we must be able to take charge and direct the flow of events and we must do that with the sympathy and cooperation of the client. The process of studying internal states and reactions requires something very different from conversation.

When you work directly with the organizers of experience, you proceed differently. Clients need to understand what the two of you are trying to do. You have to make it clear that, together, the two of you are going to study how the client creates his or her own experiences. Just doing this saves a lot of time. With more experience doing this work, you won't have to tell every client about this. You will know how to work this way and will be doing things quite automatically that will tend to bring your interactions with the client into line with this way of working. At that point in the evolution of your work, you'll only have to explain things to some clients and usually only the first time you meet. Many clients come in with ideas about how therapy proceeds; they've had other therapy experiences or they have imagined what therapy will be like. So with these clients, you've got to tell them how you intend to work.

Don't be confused about this. The client is not a problem to be solved or a story to be listened to. The client's present experience is a vivid example of how all experiences are organized and is an opportunity to study how and why experience gets organized in just that way. Experiences are grist for the mill and studying them is very different from talking about them or getting caught up in them. It's fine to be sympathetic and to feel with the client, just as long as we can step back from the details and emotional intensity of this moment and see the pattern it is part of. We must also be able to help the client to get some perspective on his experience, to study it and to reown the power that creates it. The first step towards changing oneself is a step backwards.

So, who or what does all this organizing of experience and how does he, she or it do that sort of thing? Let's first get a look at what gets organized. Second, we will discuss what does the organizing. And last, we will look at all this in relation to therapy. Consider this: a group of people with cancer are given a placebo and they're told it's a highly toxic chemotherapy drug. Over forty percent of them lose their hair. That's an example of a belief organizing physiological changes. Let's call that the output end, to include bodily change and all kinds of behavior, movement style, posture, breathing, gestures, blood flow, facial expressions, digestion, muscle tension and lots more. The list is very long. All these get organized. We use many of them in therapy: as grist for the mill, as examples of experience being organized. One can almost always bring attention to these behaviors and experience them. So, that's a whole category of experience being organized that we use in therapy: output, expression, style. A characteristic gesture is a good example. Client and therapist focus on it and study its connection to ideas, memories, and so forth, until the core organizer, a memory say, or an image, emerges into consciousness.

Okay, what about the input end? Perception is notoriously malleable. We create what we see. Perception is something taking place within the nervous system. So, how much control do we have over the creation? Are we stuck with literal translations of the various pressures, sound waves, electromagnetic fields, light waves impinging on the nervous system? Absolutely not! We select. We listen to the music and ignore the traffic in the street. Or we listen for someone's car in the drive and miss a sentence or two of what we were reading. We select. We modify, lowering light levels, numbing ourselves to the cold or heat. We fill in the blanks, imagining the faces of our friends on strangers down the street. Perception is always an act of creation. It is adding to and taking from, shaping, modifying, enhancing here, deleting there. It gets tied up with meanings, when it's influenced by needs, wants, fears, beliefs, memories, interpretation and conditioning. We organize perceptual experience, the world we create and notice, at every level.

Perceptions are also useful in therapy, again as examples of experience being organized. If I ask a client to notice what happens when I touch him or her, they can usually describe their reactions. Whatever reactions those are, they are shaped by perceptual habit and the automatic, unthinking assignment of meaning to experience. We can ask for that meaning. We can explore the way in which we created that particular experience out of the perception of touch. In doing so, we come that much closer to a conscious encounter with the memories, beliefs and expectations that are the hidden shapers of that creation. We must add that our internal world, the world that is neither input nor output but just "who we are," that is also organized. The experience of our habitual, stable, internal states, such as tensions, baseline feelings, the whole experience of self on all levels, is highly organized.

So, what are the central organizers, the important ones at the focal points of all this fervent creativity? What are we trying to get at when we do psychotherapy? We are trying to get at beliefs, images, memories, attitudes, and the important decisions we made about who we are and what type of world we're part of. We're trying to locate and look at pieces of the long ago. These events established our patterns and still control what it is possible for us to experience, feel, think and express, to this day. The central organizers are central because they organize at the deepest and most pervasive levels, affecting nearly all our experience, all the time. When you work in therapy to study how a gesture, a feeling or whatever is automatically made part of experience, you eventually come to memories, images and beliefs about who we are, what's possible for us, what type of world it is, what it wants from us and what it will give and take. These core organizers are definitions and blueprints of the most basic issues about our being in the world. They are our reference points, our measures of the self and others, with which we set our expectations, goal and limits.

When you bring one of these to consciousness, it is quickly recognized as the power figure that it is. Something like a high minister emerging from the shadows. Of course, this is what psychotherapy is all about, bringing these powerful memories and images out of the shadows and into consciousness. We all know they organize experience. That's not a secret. The skill is in bringing them into consciousness. If you try to do that through ordinary conversation, you will be hampered by the hidden rules, rules about listening, asking questions, being polite, no one being in charge of anyone else, and so forth. Effective therapy requires different rules and a different attitude towards the conversational content. It requires an experimental attitude and an openness of spirit that such an attitude implies.

Let's look at some examples of working with the organization of experience, in contrast to simply working with experience. First let's look at three roughly defined ways of interacting in therapy. One, the therapist and client engage in "ordinary conversation." That puts very wide limits on what can and will be discussed. It could be anything from a movie you saw ten years ago to something you're noticing about yourself right this minute. It could be about you or it could be about the Australian carrot crop. Personal or impersonal, present, past or future, concrete or abstract, that's the range of ordinary conversation. It is much too wide for psychotherapy. The therapist must know how to bring the client into a narrower range of more pertinent topics.

Two, there's present experience. This narrows the range. Try it with someone, sometime. The both of you just express what you are experiencing at the moment. I once did that for three hours, with two very good Gestalt therapists. The three of us staying in the here and now and talking only about our own experience. It led to one of the most beautiful times I ever had. I felt perfect, peaceful timelessness and was completely present. Okay, the therapist tries to keep the client focused within these limits, for periods of time ranging from a few seconds up to a whole session. The important experiences that emerge in those moments are then studied as examples of experience being organized by core material. That's number three, studying the organization of you know what.

Here is an example of going from one to two, that is bringing the client into present experience: The client is talking about something that got her angry last week. It's obvious from her voice that the anger is still there a little. So, the therapist says something along the lines of: seems some of that anger is still around, huh? Or, the therapist listens for a while and then asks the client to go inside and see what's happening about any of that now. The point is to get out of ordinary conversation and narrow the focus to present experience. There are any number of creative ways to do this important operation and therapists, especially Hakomi therapists, will know at least two dozen. The next examples are of working with experience without working with the organization of experience. Say the client is crying about something. The therapist uses contact statements like, "Feels sad, huh." Or the therapist asks the client to put some words to the sadness. Or the therapist touches the client or offers support. Or when a client has just noticed his/her sadness, the therapist asks, "what kind of sadness it that?" This is all about contacting, deepening and stabilizing the experience. It isn't yet going for the core. It is necessary and very important, but it isn't the heart of the matter. Here's a few examples of studying the organization. The client has been feeling some sadness and the words are something about "nobody's here for me." So, the therapist asks the client to, "notice what happens when..." and then there's the usual probe about, "I'm here for you now." Or the therapist touches the client. Some little thing we use to study reactions.

That's one big way you study the organization of experience, you set up experiments in consciousness. The therapist is saying: you get mindful, I'll say something or do something, and we will see what happens when we do that. There are two types of experiments: one where the client is passive (mindful, still) and the therapist does something, a probe, a touch, walks towards the client, closes his or her eyes, etc. In the second type, we ask the client to be active and do something like: "notice what happens when you slowly make a fist." "See what words come up when you tighten your body, the way you feel it tightening when you think of being at work."

We're not asking the client for an answer to a question. We're asking for a report on what's experienced. There's a big difference and both therapist and client should be very familiar with that difference. Experiments are for gathering information and getting reports. It isn't polite chitchat. The task at hand requires that the client report upon the results of these little experiments and that the client know that this is a part of his or her work in therapy. This task must be clear. When it isn't, therapy constantly threatens to drift back to ordinary conversation and lose the momentum needed to go deep and stay there.

Another contrast between working with experience and studying it is that when you're studying it, you can go back over something and try it again. Or you can try it a little differently; for example, the client feels some tension in his leg when you experiment with the statement: "your life belongs to you." So, you say, "let's do it again and this time notice anything else that goes on or any particular quality in the tension." That's so different from ordinary conversation. Nobody says things like, "let's say that again and you notice..." in ordinary interchanges. So, when you do things like that, you're defining the job that's being done. That's what this section has been about: defining the job of psychotherapy as the study of the organization of experience.

2

PRINCIPLES

PART 1:

SHIFTING PARADIGMS

The real is only one realization of the possible.

- Ilya Prigogine, Talk in Seattle

The fish will be the last to discover water.

- Albert Einstein

---

*(To which I would add: the fish will very likely be in deep
trouble, and a lot less water than usual, when it does. — R.K.)*

*Here are your waters and your watering place,
Drink and be whole again, beyond confusion.*

- Robert Frost, Directive

After the first nuclear explosion, Albert Einstien said, "Everything has
changed but our thinking." The incomprehensible build up of killing
power that followed makes clear how important a change in thinking is.
There have been changes in thinking before and many believe we are part of a
major shift happening right now. Such a shift, sometimes called a paradigm shift,

is at least a profound change in orientation and in the extreme a transformation of the structure of consciousness[1].

Whether we like it or not, we're all part of the changes. We are effected by the new sciences (which gave rise to the bomb, TV and computers, for example) new medicines and all the new ways to live and work and relate that were not around thirty years ago. With the world around us changing so fast, it is easy to believe a change in the structure of consciousness is under way. Or to wonder what awaits us, if it is not. If a transformation of consciousness is emerging, then something incredibly new and wonderful is happening. It could easily be the most important happening of the last three centuries.

In psychotherapy, a shift is surely under way. For one thing, there is a great variety of approaches which weren't available before. Many of these are not taught in our universities yet, nor are they sanctioned by the health care or academic establishments. For another, the context has broadened to include not only neurosis and mental illness, but teaching, organization, and personal and transpersonal growth. In all of this, allegiances have shifted, too. Many who practice psychotherapy today find philosophical ground for their work, not within the sphere of science or medicine, but in other traditions, spiritual or esoteric. For understanding the self, the old sciences, physics and chemistry, have been found wanting. The new sciences of chaos and self-organizing systems, especially as they relate to biology and physiology, are showing promise.

A Refuge for Therapists Lost. As I began to develop Hakomi, I drew, in a very intuitive way, upon whatever supports I could. I had my roots in literature, in computers and systems theory and some study of Taoism and Buddhism. I realized slowly that the work I was doing depended upon a special attitude — you might even call it a special state of consciousness. It certainly involved some very big changes in my assumptions about what I and the client were doing together. (I might as well say now, I don't like the word "client" in this context. The thesaurus offers these alternatives: buyer, customer, end user, patron... like that. I just don't know a better word, right now. Let's just think of them as, "the people who come to me".) For example, I had to shift my attitude from wanting to make something happen for the client, or making things better, to being perfectly okay if nothing happened. I realized that my agendas were getting in the way of the client's power to direct his or her own growth. My wanting to do things and to take credit for the changes didn't die easy.

My way of being with clients now is grounded in the principles. For me they are the heart of the work. They place the work in a much larger framework and they relate it to the shifting paradigm and the new structure of consciousness the paradigm will create. They guide the work, all of it, from theory, method and techniques to teaching, practice and the consciousness of the therapist. Before we meet the principles themselves, let's take a short trip through the more abstract realms of paradigm.

The Language of Paradigm

> *Now the deep structure of any given language embodies a particular syntax of perception, and the extent an individual develops the deep structure of his native language, he simultaneously learns to construct, and thus perceive, a particular type of descriptive reality, embedded, as it were, in the language structure itself. From that momentous point on... the structure of his language is the structure of his self and the limits of his world.*

- Ken Wilber, Up From Eden

The shift that's taking place is not all that easy to pin down. There are advocates of every persuasion. The dust hasn't settled. Hell, the ruckus has probably barely begun. Still, let's get a feel for it. As Wilbur is telling us, it is not just language but the syntax of perception and the structure of the self that any language (or paradigm) imposes. Our language, for example, is a subject/verb language, splitting the experiencer from the action, our logic, either/or, the logic of solid objects (but not waves). If we just list the central concepts of the "old" paradigm and contrast them with what seems to be emerging, perhaps that will suggest a framework for the principles which follow.

The Conceptual Field

In psychotherapy, as in everything we are a part of, concepts have powerful effects. The first set of concepts, the "old paradigm", creates a perceptual syntax of: inevitable isolation, unchangeable fate, cold, competitive relationships, separateness, helplessness, distance and the feeling of an uncrossable gap between my experience and yours. It motivates the search for material causes. It attempts to reduce experience to chemistry. And because it views death and destruction as inevitable, life is not a given, like order it is won through painful effort - there's no free lunch. This model fails to create any feelings of oneness, shared experience or common ground or anything greater of which we're all a part. Because the model excludes connectedness, we lose the feeling of being related to each other and the natural environment. Because we believe we are not part of them or they of us, we can destroy whole forests or whole cultures, endless species and we can poison the rivers and the oceans.

Order is held in place by effort and violence. This model does not recognize self-ordering. Nor can it motivate a search for direct knowing, without which we cannot know how much we are deeply with each other, how much we truly coexist. When only matter is real, we fail to see the value of simple contemplation.

From the present paradigm, the one we've been in and are still in, we can derive the concepts on the left. The opposite values, which it seems must be part of what the new paradigm is giving birth and rebirth to are on the right:

1. fundamental separateness	unbroken wholeness fundamental connectedness
2. absolute certitude materialism, only matter is real	uncertainty, relativity, consciousness is real, (dualism, monism)
3. exclusive, either/or logic	inclusive, both/and logic
4. mechanical and energy models linear causality	negentropic, co-evolving, information models multiple determination, non-linear causality
5. the mind/body split	mind/body integration
6. reductionist explanations	systems explanations
7. external creator-authority	self-organization, participatory authority
8. simple universal laws, fluctuations insignificant	universal complexity, disorder significant, chaos
9. dominator models, society ordered through violence	partnership models of society, ordered through family and work association
10. biology is destiny	we create our own destinies

The life of the mind is undervalued, so we become lost in a frenzy of doing. In the models of the old paradigm, the final fragmentation is the split of mind and body into separate, non-interacting realms. Mind is probably not real, they say, and even if it is, it does not and cannot influence the material world. Where does that leave psychotherapy?

Thinking in the old paradigm results in the constant fragmenting of science into separate fields, the additional partition of these fields into specialties, the separation of the scientist as person from his or her work, and the pervasive feelings of separation and isolation that grip the modern soul. There is a lack of any common ground. As Capra points out, the results of this paradigm in medicine are clear; a reductionistic view has led physicians to become so interested in the biochemistry of disease that they have completely lost sight of the whole person. It became a world full of specialists, with no room for generalists. In economics, the failure has been even more deadly. This lack of any real overview allows us to poison our world and ignore the long-range, inevitable costs, though it will cost us all dearly. This type of economics lacks ecological sense.

The old model, with its certainties and hierarchies and violence, became unworkable just when it seemed to be enjoying its greatest successes. Now that the atom can be split, and machines of untold power and cleverness and diversity populate the countryside, now we feel the loss of meaning, the threat of death and the taste of metal in the air. Now, when the war machines are suddenly capable of killing us all, there is a growing awareness that somehow we have gone quite wrong. The old model has reached its limits.

When the physicists searched for the atom with the tools of modern science, they found no solid, indestructible, absolute, eternal, separate pieces of the great machine. The "stuff of the world", as Sir James Jeans noted, "is mind stuff". A whole new view has emerged.

The New Paradigm

What they found was not absolutely anything. Newtonian physics yielded to quantum physics as the basic model. Einstein's relativity replaced the absolutist vision of time and space. Matter and energy are interchangeable. The observer is part of the equation. Modern thinking became more inclusive, less fragmented. Reductionism was seriously challenged. Mind is real, consciousness is real, not just matter. There is a new branch physics, far from equilibrium thermodynamics, developed largely by Ilya Prigogine. It is the physics of self-organizing systems, which are complex, have and maintain identities and are open and connected to their environments. This is a breakthrough in science. It connects living, biological systems to physics and shows nature to be much more than just mechanical. The whole universe may be much more alive than we had the power to imagine.

It is a participatory universe. There's no outside where you can simply stand and watch. The observer is part of the equation and the equation is full of the chatter of living. It's noisy. Certainty is gone. In its place is the knowledge that we are connected, not separate. This picture is full of juice and life. It is also more complex and allows for greater diversity and variety. Because we are more connected, it also calls for more responsibility. Nobel laureate George Wald said during the Vietnam War, we can evaluate our actions simply by asking, "Is it good for children?" Is the war good for children? Are more atomic weapons good for children? He was very sensibly introducing that simple criterion into our thinking about the war, the economy and every other area of life. He was asking us all, and scientists especially, to change their thinking, to become continuously conscious of what is now undeniable, we are all in this together.

The new paradigm is very much life-centered. As we change, concerns for all forms of life will be central to our value systems. It will come down to this, "Is it good for life?" Is it ecological? We will not survive if we continue to isolate one area of interest from another. It is disastrous to think of profits and not the cost of poisoned rivers. There's no way to fully understand an illness without understanding the person who is ill. We must become inclusive thinkers, seeing and accepting many points of view, knowing and attending to many levels and many interactions. The truth is not wholly in any one of them, but in and amongst them all. We shall learn to look beyond the selfish interests and one-pointed visions. If not, if the old thinking prevails, our small corner of the realms of life will be no more.

The New Psychotherapy

Several changes have occurred in psychotherapy over the last thirty or forty years. For one thing, we have moved from talking about experience to having experiences to studying the organization of experience; second, we have incorporated the body into psychotherapy by embracing alternative approaches such as nutrition, exercise, body work and movement, as adjuncts to the work. Particularly important are Rolfing, the Feldenkrais Method, Tai Chi, Yoga, Rolf Movement and, closer to home, the Hakomi Bodywork developed and taught by Pat Ogden of the Hakomi Institute. Lastly, we have begun to shift away from the old energy models, and are moving towards information models, like those of Bateson, NLP, Feldenkrais.

Hakomi is a part of how psychotherapy has changed and continues to change. Through the principles and in its method and technique it is a therapy based on the religious, scientific and philosophical concepts of the emerging paradigm. As much as I borrowed from older therapies, everything has been modified and adapted to accommodate the shift in perspective that was and is the principles. Hakomi is part of the transition from old to new. The five core principles are covered in detail in the following section. In these, the influence of the paradigm shift is clear and specific. We use the principles constantly to sustain and evaluate method and technique, to guide the personal development of Hakomi students, therapists and teachers and even to evaluate the progress of individual sessions. In so many ways, the work rests within the principles, like a babe in its mother's arms. Who knows, if we continue to let the principles guide us, if we stay open to what the universe is offering, who knows what we may see come to flower.

PART 2:

THE PRINCIPLES

*In the language of dynamic systems theory, the goals
injected by purposive actors into the turbulent dynamics of a
bifurcation are the stable attractors that capture the states
of the destabilized social system within a new and humanistic dynamic regime.*

- Ervin Lazlo, Evolution, The Grand Syntheses

---

*... the kind of activity which dominates the instability phase
introduces a directedness, a vector which already indicates
in which direction the new structure may be expected.*

- Erich Jantsch, The Self-Organizing Universe

---

*In the kingdom of the blind, the one-eyed
man is king.*

- Michael Apostelius, Proverbs

The principles are the most immediate and important part of the therapist's knowledge. We speak of therapists or students as "working (or not
working) within the principles". To work within the principles is to
incorporate the principles as an unconscious base for one's therapeutic approach
and to act continuously out of that particular mind set. When I work with people,
I am working from a part of myself that knows and lives by the principles. It feels
like an altered state of consciousness.

Being in the principles — which by the way, takes no effort at all once you
surrender to them — I would argue, does almost all the work. The principles are
part of an emotional attitude which appreciates the other's freedom and aliveness
and part of a consciousness that keenly follows all that the other is expressing.
Such consciousness and emotional attitude are felt by the deeper parts of the other,
earning the cooperation of the unconscious. With that, the work becomes
infinitely easier. Being without the principles is like working blind.

Most people who come to study Hakomi already have a kindred feeling
towards the work. They say after hearing about it or seeing it, "I knew it was

right." "I work that way myself; I just didn't have words for it." "It felt like something I already knew." They are relating mostly to the principles. They really don't know the method or the techniques, but something feels good to them, something feels familiar. It is their appreciation of the principles in action. For these people, learning the work will be easy and a joy.

We study the principles in the training, learning to incorporate each one as a basic part of our work. We use them and practice them and finally, we make them a fundamental aspect of our lives. Being in the principles frees us to be comfortable and creative. As they become incorporated, we use them without effort or thought. We are comfortable that whatever we do will help rather than harm. That feeling frees us to be creative. Therapy is not just a job. An idea like that says very little about the therapist as an instrument or an artist or a healer. Therapy is healing. Knowledge of the principles grounds us in several, potent traditions and unlocks our potential to be helpful to others.

Science is not complete, especially in the realms of the mind. A psychotherapy confined by an image of itself as a scientific endeavor will also be incomplete. Our therapy is not simply method and technique, at the heart of it all is the spirit of the work.

Organicity: Living Systems

> *Living things are called organisms because of the overriding importance of organization, and each part of the pattern somehow contains the information as to what it is in relation to the whole.*

- Robert O. Becker, The Body Electric

> *In wild nature there is no disorder: no plant in the almost endless mosaics of micro and macro communities is really out of place.*

- Gary Snyder, Good, Wild, Sacred

> *This circularity, this connection between action and experience, this inseparability between a particular way of being and the way the world appears to us, tells us that... every act of knowing brings forth a world.*

- Humberto Maturana and Francesco Varela, The Tree of Knowledge

*I have been trying to imagine a framework for the origin of
life, guided by a personal philosophy which considers the
primal characteristics of life to be homeostasis rather than
replication, diversity rather than uniformity, the flexibility of
the cell rather than the tyranny of the gene, the error
tolerance of the whole rather than the precision of the parts.*

*... the qualitative features which I consider essential:
looseness of structure and tolerance of errors.*

*Tolerance for junk is one of life's most essential
characteristics.*

- Freeman Dyson, Infinite in All Directions

Life is one damn thing after another.

- Mark Twain

Psychotherapy is healing and healing only happens to living organisms. You
can fix a car or a bookcase, you can repair a television set or a computer — but
you don't heal them. And they don't heal themselves. Only living systems heal;
they don't get fixed or repaired or anything like that. An MD can set a fracture,
but he cannot heal it. He must wait and see if it will heal. He can help, but he
cannot heal. Healing is an act of self-recreation. One being cannot heal another.
The other can only help or hinder. The organicity principle places the locus of
healing and control within the client and the client-therapist relationship. The
client's growth and unfolding, his or her answers and resolutions, completions
and new directions, are all within. The therapist is there to help manage the
process through which the client goes there and gets them.

To understand and work from this perspective, we must be clear about the
difference between living systems and non-living systems. Organicity refers to
the process dynamics of self-organization — the internally directed creation,
maintenance and evolution of living systems. Recent systems theory, theoretical
biology and a new physics have emerged which attempt to define and explain this
difference. This new work is based in great part on Ilya Prigogine's work with
dissipative structures[2] on the concepts of autopoeisis, developed by Maturana and
Varella[3] and on the dynamics of self-organization, developed by modern systems
theorists, in particular, Erich Jantsch and Ervin Lazlo[4]. The spiritual tradition that
speaks most clearly to this principle is Taoism[5].

This new theory of living systems is a lusty affirmation of personal freedom and the natural intelligence of all life. Living systems self-organize, self-create, self-maintain, and in many ways, direct their own evolution. Life is its own authority. Life is creative; it tends to jump around and come up with new ways to do things. Unlike machines, living beings get bored[6]. This exuberance of living systems is balanced by their incredible sensitivity to their surroundings. Living systems are by their very natures: participatory and interactive. All living systems must be open to their environment. They must import energy, matter and information and they must export or dissipate entropy (noise, waste and disorder). Living is continuous exchange and this exchange is a natural, physical process. Life is not an accident nor is it probable that we are alone in the universe. By the very fact of their existence, all beings belong.

When you embrace the organicity principle, you look for and follow natural processes. You do not impose a structure or an agenda on the process, but you seek the sources of movement and growth and support these. It is as simple as leaving the client time, after every interaction, to make the next move, to pursue his or her interests and direction — instead of, for example, asking a question about something that interests you. It is very easy, in a position of "authority" like therapist, to take control and run the whole session. In Hakomi, we go as far as supporting the defenses, those habits of the client which helps him or her manage important experiences. Recognizing that organic systems have their own paths and purposes and will resist attempts to force them in directions they don't want to go, we have found a way to go with the defenses that supports rather than prevents growth. Taking over is the technique, but it is the attitude of acceptance of the other's self-direction that sets the stage.

In general, the principle of organicity asserts our respect for life and our faith in the healing power of the individual. It creates an atmosphere of freedom, self-determination and responsibility for the client and it allows the therapist to act and feel more like a healer than a mechanic. It also works hand in hand with the next two principles, mindfulness, which replaces physical effort as the source of change, and nonviolence, which calls the other, "partner".

Mindfulness: The Path of Consciousness

If you can pour a cup of tea right, you can do anything.

- Gurdjieff

*There's two ways to wash the dishes. You can wash the
dishes in order to clean the dishes or you can wash the
dishes in order to wash the dishes.*

- Thich Nhat Hanh, The Miracle of Mindfulness

---

*If, in ordinary life, mindfulness, or attention, is directed to
any object, it is rarely sustained long enough for the
purpose of factual observation. Generally, it is followed
immediately by emotional reaction, discriminative thought,
reflection, purposeful action.*

- Nyanoponika, The Power of Mindfulness

Mindfulness is both a principle and a state of consciousness. As a principle, it is part of the meditative and contemplative traditions. For me, Buddhism especially is important. As an attitude which the therapist holds, it speaks of a preference for the path of consciousness. It declares its faith by taking the time to simply study experience before doing anything about it. J.P. Morgan once said, "All else being equal, I choose the man who tastes his food before he salts it." Mindfulness begins like that, with a preference for tasting over doing, a preference for noticing, how one is being touched and moved in consciousness, how one is organizing one's experience. Mindfulness is part of a tradition that recognizes the reality of consciousness, either as equally real or more real than matter. It also recognizes organicity, openness and sensitivity, and it allows the inner wisdom of the other to create change through awareness rather than effort.

As we use mindfulness in Hakomi, it might be called assisted meditation. In therapy, its greatest effect is simply staying with experience longer, before following "immediately by emotional reaction, discriminative thought, reflection, purposeful action." It is a matter of staying a little longer, gathering more information and allowing things to happen by themselves. Highly complex, living systems like we humans, organize our perceptions and actions around core images and beliefs. In ordinary consciousness, going about the daily business of life, these core beliefs exert control without our being conscious of their influence. They function in the background, unnoticed. One of the main goals of the therapeutic process is to bring this organizing material into consciousness, to study it and understand it. Mindfulness, as a state of consciousness, is the tool we use.

As a state of consciousness, mindfulness has the following characteristics: it is focused on present experience, traditionally, the contents of consciousness. We can't be mindful of the past; we know only that we are remembering the past, because that remembering takes place in the present. The route to mindfulness is present-centered attention. Mindfulness is "willfully passive". We deliberately decide to observe present experience without interfering with it. This receptive attitude, if exercised for only a few moments at a time, can yield rich insights. Finally, attention during mindfulness is, for the most part, turned inward. We can however allow external influences to be part of the present experience we are noticing. When we do this deliberately in therapy, we do it to evoke experiences that we will later process. The hope is that by bringing these experiences into consciousness we will be able in some way to transcend them, to know them, to complete them and to move on.

Nonviolence: Reverence for Life

> *The rush and pressure of modern life are a form, perhaps the most common form, of its innate violence. To allow oneself to be carried away by a multitude of conflicting concerns, to surrender to too many demands, to commit oneself to many projects, to want to help in everything is to succumb to violence. The frenzy of the activist neutralizes work for peace. It destroys the fruitfulness of work, because it kills the root of inner wisdom which makes work fruitful.*

- Thomas Merton

> *... The ideal posture is obtained not by doing something to oneself, but by literally <u>doing nothing</u>, that is, by eliminating all acts of voluntary origin due to motivations other than standing that have become automatic and are now part and parcel of the personal acture of the situation of standing.*

- Moshe Feldenkrais, The Potent Self

> *Consequently: he who wants to have right without wrong, order without disorder, does not understand the principles of heaven and earth. He does not know how things hang together.*

- Chuang Tzu, Great and Small

Nonviolence is a practical recognition of organicity. It is a policy of going with the grain, of staying with what is natural, because that's what works. Going against the grain, using force against a living system is asking for resistance. In Taoism, there is the principle of Mutual Arising. It refers to opposites being necessary. For example, the day you were born, your death was possible. Or, keep eating those free salty peanuts, you're going to order another beer. In therapy it is: if you use violence, you will get resistance.

Violence in therapy is very subtle. It is not that obvious to people raised with the models of authority common to our culture. When someone simply assumes they know what is best for others, you have violence. You have the opposite of organicity. When therapists ask questions to gather information for themselves, often interrupting the client to do so, that's violence, and it breeds resistance. The client may sit through the hour and go through the motions, but something inside them takes offense and begins to resist. Violence in therapy is not just deliberate, physical harm. It is a failure to accept the whole person who is client, a person with his own story, her own ideas, images, needs, wishes, capacities, pace. Violence is being too much stuck in yourself and your own agenda to really be healing for another.

Nonviolence is born of an attitude of acceptance and an active attention to the way events naturally unfold. It works hand in hand with mindfulness, which helps us to understand without interfering. It takes a long time to learn. It is of course a central tenet in both Buddhism and Christianity, each with long traditions and much literature[7].

In the therapy, we see nonviolence operating in several ways. One important way is our work with what are called, "defenses". (Sounds like we may have to attack.) I prefer to call those same behaviors, "managing experience". In speaking of these behaviors as defensive, our attitudes around force and authority are revealed and an image is conjured of the client getting in the therapist's way. In Hakomi, we do not oppose the client's efforts to manage his or her experience. We support these in an effort to give the client a safe and controlled way to explore the experiences more deeply and completely. Any attempt to oppose such management meets with resistance anyway and the work becomes effortful and more painful than it need be. The client's style of management is after all the client's best efforts to deal with real pain and fear in many situations. This style is an old and valuable part of the client's tools for meeting his or her world. Our support for these shows a deep respect for the whole person.

A second way nonviolence operates is by placing the emphasis on experience rather than advice or interpretation. We are not there to solve problems, or to tell the client who he or she is. Our responsibility is to help the client reach certain key experiences, experiences the client has not had before, experiences that teach the client what is possible for her or him. By gaining the cooperation of the unconscious and following and supporting the client's own pace and process, we create a situation where those experiences that need and want to happen have their natural place. When we simply support, the client does the work he or she has to do and it is a sign of our success that client takes the credit, which they well deserve, for the doing.

Mind-Body Holism

> *... The implication of these findings is that there may be a 55% placebo response from many, if not all, healing procedures. Such a consistent degree of placebo response also suggests there is a common underlying mechanism or process that accounts for mind-body communication and healing, regardless of the problem, symptom or disease.*

- Ernest Rossi, The Psychobiology of Mind-Body Healing

> *... In the final analyses, the ability of the human nervous system to make individual patterns, or the ability to learn from personal experience, is so much greater in man that we can consider it as a new quality.*

- Moshe Feldenkrais, The Potent Self

Holism is a recognition of complexity and the inherent unpredictability of the whole by the parts. It is the recognition of the influence of each aspect of living on all the others. It sees patterns and interactions and nonlinear influences. Good examples are acupuncture and the theories of self-organizing systems[8]. Mind and body are such a system.

Mind and body influence one another. They interact. This principle puts Hakomi Therapy in the camp of the mind-body interactionists[9]. My particular interest is in the influence deeply held beliefs, guiding images and significant, early memories have on behavior, body structure and all levels of physiology, from cellular metabolism and the strength of the immune system, to blood flow and the distribution of heat and muscle tone in the body, to the expression of these beliefs in posture, movement, gesture and facial expression. There are of course influences that body has on mind — from the inheritance of talents and disposi-tions to the moods that are part of having a diseased liver. These influences are often circular and complexly determined through the operations of feedback loops. We will examine some of these loops when we look at how behavior patterns and belief systems stabilize each other, but as this book is about changing core beliefs and images in order to change experience, I focus primarily on mind influencing body.

In therapy, we attempt to work constantly at the "mind-body interface". We work with the interaction of belief and experience, image and emotion. Sometimes we work by focusing attention on bodily experience and ask for meaning or belief. Sometimes we focus attention on belief or meaning and study the experiences evoked. We alternate one direction with the other, constantly crossing and staying as close as possible to the mind-body interface.

Unity: A Participatory Universe

This type of consciousness — what I shall refer to in this book as "participatory consciousness" — involves merger, or identification, with one's surroundings, and bespeaks a psychic wholeness that has long since passed from the scene.

- Morris Berman, The Reenchantment Of The World

We deal with the products of the world's tendency to generate parts out of wholes made up of units connected together by communication. It is this that makes the body a living thing, which acts as if it had a mind — which indeed it does.

- Gregory Bateson

"A psychic wholeness that has long since passed from the scene", Morris Berman's phrase. I think of that wholeness when I see a newborn infant or, as happened last week, a Maori person sang a Maori parting song as a group we were in was ending. He sang about going away over the sea. Parting and traveling long distances, for the Maori, are always associated with the sea. They are an island culture. As he sang, I could feel his love and knowledge of the sea. I felt like we were there, on the sea, sailing away. That feeling was as real as the room we were in. This singer's psychic wholeness certainly hadn't passed from the scene — it created the scene, it allowed him to bring sea and sky, his people and his whole world with him, because they were him. His was a participatory universe. He was his family, his people and the natural world around him in a way that we have simply lost. He belonged to this world and was comfortable in it in a way we never have been.

Unity is about belonging, being part of, about hearing and being heard. Many therapies take integration and harmony as major concerns. The feldenkrais method, Rolfing, osteopathy, acupuncture, gestalt are examples. Whether we are talking about people joining to be a family, muscles joining to create movement, organs harmonizing in a healthy body, or thoughts, ideas, beliefs, impulses, plans, feelings, memories joining to become a single self, all these systems speak about unity and integration. We study such systems by exploring the ways in which they enable and support communication among their parts and conversely, how they collapse, suffer and die as communication breaks down and stops.

Eastern religious tradition has it that unity is real and the notion that we are separate entities is illusion. The primary and most destructive illusion is the false distinction between self and other. "Self" here doesn't even mean you're a person or a body or any thing like that. It means you perceive and live a basic separateness. This is the primal lie. You can compare the movement from unity to duality to that from a holographic wave front to images of separate objects. A hologram is a network of wave patterns, like ripples on a lake during the rain. You have to decode the patterns if you wish to perceive separate objects. You have to take this intermingling, integrating, holographic universe and split it into separate "selves" and "others." For all this you need encoders. Well, according to Karl Pribram, all the senses, including touch, are encoders. The East has always known that the senses lie. We see each other as separate objects because we see through our eyes and because we have learned to think of our selves and others in that way. The unencumbered heart sees differently.

We split our universe at several levels. Ken Wilbur covers this in great detail[10]. The big break comes when we decide that we are separate. We further separate ourselves into minds and bodies; the mind/body split. This particular level has been the focus of intense study, religious practice and endless speculation. Finally, not only do we split mind and body, but mind itself splits into pieces. Our capacity to experience is severely stunted when we fracture the mind/body unity. Then the mind splits into "me" and "not me". Wholeness, integrity, harmony are lost at each level. Jung called the parts of the mind "shadow" and "persona," the hidden and the mask. Neither is real. We separate into the parts we own and take responsibility for and those we don't. We're not consciously saying this is me and that is not me. We don't hear those other parts; we don't listen to them, look at them or feel them. We actively avoid them.

Psychotherapists work to get parts communicating, whether it's members of a family, the body and the mind or parts of mind. It's an art, full of high skills, to coax those parts out of hiding, to help them speak openly and directly, to help someone do that. I think Gestalt Therapy is especially good at that. Gestalt Therapists work in the language of drama and theater. They work with the interaction of the parts we play. Gestalt Therapy is all about parts and wholes. In the hot seat, you create a dialogue. You talk to a projection of some part of yourself, a part you don't want to own, a part you have pushed away. In this dialogue, these parts start to communicate again. That's the most important thing about the process; it gets communication going again. It's not just the dialogue that's significant, it's the process itself. Perls has faith (and so do I) that if you can get those parts communicating again, they may resolve their differences and come to harmony. It's a sure thing they won't if they don't communicate. When the dialog takes place within a context of safety and concern, as in healing relationship, the chances for integration are much greater.

This drive to unite is the healing force. This process of communication, organizes parts into wholes. That's the healing. "The psyche spontaneously reorganizes," to quote Ken Wilbur. The nervous system spontaneously reorganizes, according to Feldenkrais. Given a communication among the parts involved in movement, they will spontaneously integrate around the most effortless functioning. The extraneous drops away. Health is a natural result of the attention each part gives to the others. This is the faith that healers have.

In therapy, we attempt to establish and enhance communication between conscious and unconscious, and between mind and body. In using mindfulness, we create opportunities which allows the unconscious a clear chance to express and be seen, heard and felt. In our focus on the mind-body interface, we work to create channels of communication between them. When we work with the child, we are often hearing from a part that has long been suppressed and silent. When the client comes to insight, meaning and self-acceptance, again it is one part understanding or accepting another.

The unity principle states that the universe is fundamentally a web of relationships in which all aspects and components are inseparable from the whole and do not exist in isolation. This contrasts sharply with the Atomistic and Newtonian visions of indestructible, indivisible, isolated bits of matter afloat in an otherwise absolutely empty container called "space." The implications for the type of consciousness created by these contrasting visions of reality concern every level of being and living.

We embrace unity when we bring attention to aspects of ourselves and others that are in isolation and conflict. We embrace it when our way is acceptance and curiosity; when our goal is to bring together all aspects of the person: mind/mind, mind/body and self/universe; when we know as part of our being that we are connected, to each other and this world. That knowing is the healing power of this work.

PART 3:
THE BATESON PROPOSITIONS

I n *Mind and Nature,* Gregory Bateson says that there are certain qualities, certain characteristics of any system that can be said to have mind. Bateson describes these qualities through a set of propositions. He finds that this same set of propositions applies both to the human mind and to nature. Nature, as Bateson defines it, has mind. Nature acts intelligently. If you look at evolution, it's an intelligent process — clever, strategic. So are ecological systems. I want to discuss Bateson's propositions and their similarity to the Hakomi principles.

Let's go over Bateson's set of six propositions to describe any system that has mind. The first one is that minds are made up of parts organized into wholes. Parts into wholes, the unity principle. If you just think about parts into wholes for a couple of days, you'll see that an incredible number of systems — families, human organs, football teams — all exhibit that quality. Parts into wholes. Atoms into molecules. Stars into galaxies. This is also about organicity and self-organizing systems.

The second proposition: the parts communicate. The parts organize into wholes through communication and information. We are not dealing with energy, but information. Osteopathic medicine is an example of an information model. Osteopathy is based on the notion that a disease is a condition where messages are not getting from one part of your body to another. If you are ill, you have a communications problem. In osteopathy, the spine is the main channel for messages. When an osteopath adjusts the spine, he or she is trying to get the parts of the body to communicate better. Even germ theory can be seen as an information flow model: some part of the immune system isn't detecting germs or isn't communicating about them to the right parties. The techniques we use in Hakomi — probes, witnessing, taking over — are all ways of getting information about how we organize ourselves. We could say that one part of ourselves is learning to communicate with another. Parts into wholes through communication and information.

There is a common statement of faith in all healing systems based on communication. Straighten the spine to help the messages get back and forth and system function will improve. It is the faith that with open, part to part communication, the system will self-correct. If you are stuck. the strategy is: hang out, use awareness and curiosity, get clear information moving between the parts and you'll get an automatic, spontaneous resolution and improvement in function. In Hakomi, we study and work with precisely those habits which interfere with gathering information and spontaneous reorganization. We talk about creating "options at the barriers".

The capacity to self-correct (to heal) is a quality of all living systems. If you move with awareness, function improves "spontaneously." The organism knows how to integrate. Reorganization happens because the parts are communicating again. The neck muscles know what the pelvis is doing. They are no longer isolated. They are in relationship. They are resonant. They start to operate as a whole. Since such integration is in the best interests of the organism, the impulse towards becoming whole is strong and present in all living systems. The parts communicate — Bateson's second proposition.

The third proposition states that energy is collateral. Information is the important thing. What is important about minds is not the way they process energy; it's how they process information. Of course, you've got to have some energy. The kind doesn't matter. We deal with information. The system has to have energy, but that is not as significant as what type of mind is using that energy. A system can have a lot of energy and not much mind. Think of atom bombs! The muscles are all directed by nerves. The mind is primary. Given lots or little energy, it is still the mind which will direct how that energy is used.

We may be coming out of our energy-centered age. And out of the type of consciousness that's focused on power, the kind that believes there's just so much to go around. Perhaps the dream of endless free energy will come true. If it is about energy and energy is limited, the focus on power and separation will remain. If I give you one of my hamburgers or a gallon of my gasoline, I have less. That's the nature of thinking in terms of energy. It's either/or thinking. Either I have that gasoline or you do. But if we're talking about information, the situation is entirely different. When I tell you something, I still know it. After I've told you, we both know it. Both/and. Both you and me. On a practical level, that's the nature of information. It's very hard to own information. Ask the guys who want to protect records and video tapes from being copied. Unlike matter and energy, a given piece of information can be in two places at once. I don't lose it just because I give it to you. A different type of consciousness evolves when mind and information are primary and energy and force, secondary.

The first computer, Von Neumann's, had 18,000 electron tubes. It filled a huge room with electronic equipment, and it used 140,000 watts. In that system, energy was significant (particularly if you were paying the electric bill). I bought a computer this year that has the equivalent of over a million electron tubes and it burns one quarter of a watt. It fits in a space smaller than a typewriter. The energy required is no big deal and its capacity for processing information boggles the mind. Minds are information systems. If you're going to study the organization of mind, energy is collateral. Psychotherapy is an information-oriented process. It's true, the human energy system is very complex and it's important to keep it tuned up, but if you're going to think about how people organize their experience, the operations of mind are your priorities.

Bateson's fourth proposition is this: all systems that exhibit mind can only be described by using circular or more complex determination. If you are going to work with people, you had better be ready to celebrate complexity. You'd better love diversity and be very happy with uncertainty. Systems with mind are more complex than simple, linear systems[11]. They are not like cue balls, where this one hits that one and that one and that one. You cannot trace the workings of mind that way. Systems with mind have feedback loops. They are non-linear, iterative, creative, diverse. They have parts that communicate, that talk back and forth. You can't just say; "Well, if I push here, then the whole thing will go like so." It's not that simple. A system with mind has it's own, internal organization. It will adjust to what you do. You may not know what type of adjustment it's going to make, which is why it's so difficult to describe how any particular mind operates.

Proposition five says that <u>information is coded. You're taking your experi-</u><u>ence and you're organizing it</u>. That's what's meant by coding. There are no pictures in the brain; rather, the eye encodes the visual information that reaches it into nerve impulses. At some levels encoding is fixed; at other levels, you can change the way you encode your experience. In psychotherapy, we're interested in high-level coding, such as our theories about ourselves and about the world. A proposition like "I have to earn people's approval and love" organizes a lot of experience. People who are performance-oriented, who are not able to slow down and rest, often put that transformation on their experience. They are shaping their lives, judgments and decisions around it. If somebody says, "You did a good job," it can have a big effect on them. They also have muscle habits which deal with the ideas and thoughts around that issue. They mobilize their muscles for action and their minds are sharply focused on the tasks to be completed. So this proposition tells us that we organize our experience and, on a higher level, it implies that we can change the way we organize our experience.

The sixth proposition states that these <u>organizations are in some type of</u> <u>hierarchy</u>. Bateson uses Bertrand Russell's theory of logical types. You can write on a blackboard a statement such as this: "This blackboard has nothing on it." Such a statement, according to Russell, doesn't make any sense. A statement about the blackboard is a different order of business from being the blackboard; it's a different logical type. These logical types come into play in living systems because we're dealing with levels of organization. The whole self is a higher logical type than either mind or body. A whole mind is a higher logical type than conscious or unconscious. <u>These systems have logical levels</u>. It's important not to confuse one level with the other. <u>You are not your thoughts,</u> you are not your body. <u>You're all this and more than this</u>. <u>At some level you are the whole</u> universe.

It is much more important to understand and embrace the principles than it is to learn techniques. Techniques will emerge spontaneously from a knowledge of the principles. It's more important to have the feel of the work, than to have the theory. We need both, but the feeling is primary. The emotional attitude, the basic psychological orientation of the therapist is primary. The principles are simple, but they're not something people hurry to embrace; mindfulness and nonviolence are not most people's immediate concerns; more often we're energy oriented. In the principles, there's the power to learn, to grow and change, to evolve and ultimately, to be free. With mindfulness, change comes without much effort. Still, we often seem to prefer effort. Of course, struggle has the power to make heroes of us. Violence and heroism are usually parts of the same story.

"The great way is not difficult for those who have no preferences." No preferences. No fighting with what simply is. This Zen attitude is basic to both mindfulness and nonviolence. The body mobilizes to deal with situations as the mind understands them. In this way the body reflects mental life. Our understanding, dispositions, expectations and plans all affect the body. When you have expectations, your body prepares to act accordingly. In your anger, when you are so disposed, you will surely find something to be angry about.

If you have preferences, you also mobilize your body. If you have desires, if you want something to happen in a certain way, if you are emotionally attached to the outcomes of your efforts and choices, your body will participate. You can't even want something strongly without your body "clutching" as you think of it. If you let yourself, even for a moment, feel a mood of wanting, longing, you'll notice that your body tenses. Like a big hand, the body grasps at the desired outcome. The person without preferences doesn't hold on this way. Without preferences, there is no violence to the body, no clutching with desire. The person without preferences accepts what is. In that yielding, there is no effort and no violence. When you study and understand your body tensions, you learn a great deal about your core beliefs. For example, if I usually have my eyes wide open and my shoulders up around my neck, my beliefs probably have to do with how dangerous the world is. A good observer can "see" those fears in me. I can see them myself when I am mindful.

We need mindfulness to drop preferences, because you can't even know your preferences without mindfulness. Without mindfulness, you won't be in touch with your beliefs and dispositions. Without paying attention, without awareness, you will be operating out of habit, out of reaction and automatic behaviors. You will be moving perhaps, getting things done, but you won't be learning, changing, growing and becoming freer. If you are not mindful, you cannot know or change yourself. Without observing and thinking about and knowing yourself simply as you are, you can't transform. Only when you know what your core beliefs are can you challenge them. Only when "you know what you're doing, can you do what you want." Until you understand how your beliefs keep you going, you won't be able to stop. You are close to freedom when you know your deepest beliefs about yourself and the words that express those beliefs are true and precise. Mindful-

ness clarifies. The more enlightened among us have given up childish preferences. They have looked into their own minds and yielded everything which does
violence to life and truth. But, to give up preferences, you must first know you
have them and what they are.

Notes for Chapter 2.

1. See Georg Feuerstein's, *Structures of Consciousness*. Lower Lake, Calif.:
Integral Publishing, 1987.
2. See Ilya Prigogine and Iasbelle Stenger's, *Order Out of Chaos*. New York:
Bantam Books, 1984.
3. See Humberto Maturana and Francisco Varela's, *The Tree of Knowledge*.
Boston: Shambhala Publications, Inc., 1987
4. Erich Jantsch, *The Self-Organizing Universe*. Oxford: Pergamon Press, 1980,
and Irwin Lazlo, Evolution: The Grand Synthesis. Boston: Shambhala Publication, Inc., 1987.
5. There are any number of translations of the Tao Te Ching, by Lao Tzu. Chuang
Tzu is another Taoist figure and a good book about him is *When the Shoe Fits*, by
Bhagwan Shree Rajneesh.
6. Douglas Hofstaeder cites this as the difference between machines and living
beings, "machines don't get bored".
7. Some books: Kalu Rimpoche, *The Dharma*. Albany: State University of New
York Press, 1986. And, Nyanaponica Thera, *The Vision of Dhama*. York Beach,
Maine: Samuel Wiser, Inc., 1986.
8. See Fritjof Capra's, *The Turning Point*. Boston: Beacon Press, Inc., 1982.
9. *The Self and Its Brain* by Karl Popper and John Eccles is a good book on the
interaction of mind and body, emphasizing "top-down causality", a phrase that
reductionists don't quite get.
10. See Ken Wilbur's, *The Spectrum of Consciousness*. Boulder, CO: Shambala,
1977
11. "There are no systems in biology where more is better all the time." That's
another Bateson quote.

3

PEOPLE

*The basic reason for strong convergence, prosaic as it may
seem, is simply that some ways of making a living impose
exacting criteria of form and function on any organism
playing the role.*

- Stephen Jay Gould, Ever Since Darwin

---

*These abstract forms are optimal solutions for common
problems."*

- D'arcy Thompson, On Growth and Form

To [Wilhelm] *Reich, dreams were no longer the cornerstones
of therapy. The manner in which the patient comes to the
treatment, his politeness or stubbornness, his mode of speech,
his dress, the style and firmness of his handshake were all
records of character. And character is real, it can be treated.
Reich directed attention to this and away from the complica-
tion of content and free association, which engage and
distract the interest of the regular analyst.*

*Since the Freudian unconscious was basically latent sensa-
tions and impulses in the body itself, Reich saw no predomi-
nant need to go back in time to the traumatic moment or
origin of the condition. He wrote "The entire world of past*

> *experience (is) embodied in the present in the form of char-*
> *acter attitudes. A person's character is the fractional sum*
> *total of all past experiences."*
>
> *The doctor does not need to reconstruct a traumatic*
> *moment; the traumatic moment continues to exist in every*
> *breath the patient takes, in every gesture he makes.*
>
> - Richard Grossinger, Planet Medicine

C entral to a holistic approach to the study of people is the notion that human activity is "multipli-determined." Many different influences combine in the development and maintenance of the patterns we study in psychotherapy. The search for one great traumatic event, so popular in movies about psychotherapy, doesn't happen that often in therapy. What truly helps a person is to realize and understand whole patterns and the beliefs, feelings, images and memories the patterns are influenced by. We call these patterns *character* or *character strategies*. It is wise to remember that these are "abstract forms" and simplifications. There are no characters out there in the real world, there are only people. The patterns, limited in number and similar from person to person, reflect similar issues and common needs and experiences. This commonality should not distract us from the truth that each individual is unique and must be treated so[1]. Understanding patterns helps us by making complex individual lives expressions of common roots. A study of character strategies gives us a general feel for people, how they handle their daily tasks and encounters with others, how they learned to do it that way, what kinds of events and memories, feelings and beliefs organize their life strategies.

Character patterns are the result of an ongoing interaction of the growing child with its physical/emotional environment. These patterns and strategies can be seen as strengths developed by the child. In this light, character is more correctly seen as function rather than malfunction. But, a strength developed to the point of imbalance is also a weakness and every function overly developed in one direction leaves another direction undeveloped. For example, the strength some people develop to bear up under difficult conditions may leave those same people little sense of joy and lightness. In one of the patterns we study — the burdened-enduring pattern — the over developed strength of bearing up under blame leads to difficulties in taking responsibility and action.

We can think about character patterns in many different ways: as strengths or weaknesses, function or malfunction; as reflections of the strategies other creatures use (what I'm calling bio-strategies); as adjustment processes to the particular stress of information overload[2]; and in a number of other ways. My personal preference is to look at character as strategy.

Bio-Strategies

On the coasts of California, small, silvery grunion, come up on the beaches by the thousands to lay and fertilize their eggs. They always come at the time of the full moon, when the tide is highest and the eggs can remain undisturbed in the sand till the next high tide, some ten days later. The endless cycles of the sea have shaped the grunion to the tides. We could call this way of using the tide a grunion strategy. It is strategic in the sense that it is purposeful and clever. Of course, this seeming purpose is not the result of thinking and planning. It only seems so. It is part of the play of action and interaction that the species grunion has engaged in. So, there is a beautiful harmony played out, as if a key had been made for just this lock that the moon has upon the oceans. It is this intricate fitting together of organism and environment that suggests strategy and purpose. All we know of character patterns also suggests a beautiful and intricate fit that each person makes with his or her felt emotional and psychological environment. The management of experience, the use of defenses, habits, personal myths[3] and styles, all make sense as strategy. So, we talk now of character and bio-strategies.

Animals species have grown into ways of dealing with their worlds that seem much like the patterns we call character. My favorite example is the strategy of deception. Animals use a whole array of disguises and deceptive colorations. Some species enhance their ability to survive by looking like something or somebody they are not, like the non-poisonous snakes and caterpillars that look very much like the poisonous ones. Deception is the main strategy of a pattern we call tough-generous or charming-seductive, similar to Lowen's narcissistic-psychopathic dimension[4]. Looking dangerous or innocent (or important, or confident, or relaxed) when you're not really that way or not feeling that way, is the key strategy of the tough-generous.

Take birds and moths. Some moths fool birds by having big round dark spots on their wings that look like a larger animal's eyes. Fooling others, especially by making them perceive you as bigger, stronger, dangerous, more intelligent, richer, or more important than you are is a common strategy and one that can be a person's basic character pattern. The opposite approach, looking harmless and friendly when you are neither, can also be a life-long deception strategy. Animals like the angler fish, which has an enticing looking little tongue and a very big mouth, and humans like the camouflaged hunter who lies in wait for the unsuspecting, use this strategy. There is a connection here to the burdened-enduring pattern. Both play innocent. With the tough-generous or charming-seductive, this innocence is central to the strategy, with the burdened-enduring, it is secondary, an outer reflection of an inner feeling of too much responsibility. Some other bio-strategies are: (1) freezing, playing dead, suppressing movement and keeping a low profile — these are the bio-strategies of the hunted and the trapped; (2) looking weak and needy, an extension of infantile characteristics and a time when the young need to be fed and kept safe and warm by the parenting ones. From baby seals to little kangaroos, from the newly hatched to the larvae of bees, all are kept and cared for. (3) The burdened-enduring, like turtles and clams, build a strong, insensitive shell and let you wear yourself out using force on them. (4) The expressive-clinging, like the great whooping cranes whose loud cries announce their coming, need to be noticed and attended to. They usually make a fuss or have something exciting to share — something that will get and hold attention. Of course, these strategies work. When the child needed attention, from some over focused parent perhaps, he or she got louder or sicker or more destructive or whatever it took to get attention from that absorbed parent. So, whoop they did and whoop worked. Just as deception in the tough-generous pattern worked. (5) The industrious-overfocused seems to me like a bulldog whose "dogged" persistence wins the day when he chomps on some bull's nose and just hangs on until the game's up. The strategy is persistence.

Character As Strategy

Character processes are strategies. A defense is a general way of dealing with the world, a way of managing one's experience. People are creative and we find various strategies within one person. That allows us to hold several theories about a person without having to try to decide what "type" he or she is. A person can be several, all at once. We can stop beating our heads on the wall trying to figure out which type we really are or which type somebody else really is. We are diverse and clever and complex. We don't have to reduce people to types. Any systematic description of human behavior can be pertinent and useful to us. Anything may illuminate the patterns we encounter. We don't have to argue about which is the right description. We're not looking for causes here; we're looking for systems and consistencies. It's not a question of which one is true. It's a question of how much can I learn from each. Knowing this changes the attitude and consciousness of the therapist. In seeing character as strategy, we link core material to its expression as reactions to perceived situations.

Character strategies are organized, habitual patterns of reaction. They are long used responses to real or perceived stress or to goals, needs and wishes. Real stress, like chronic pain or poverty, as crucial as they are, are not that important, for our purposes. What is important is beliefs, expectations, unresolved emotions, uncertainties about oneself and one's relation to others, in other words, the organization of experience by core material.

The Eight Major Strategies Used in Hakomi[5]

1. sensitive/withdrawn	minimize self-expression/contact with others. take refuge in thought and fantasy.
2. dependent/endearing	seek support by acting childlike.
3. self-reliant/ independent	mobilize self-support and rely on oneself. seek challenges.
4. deceptive 1 tough/generous	hide your weakness, insecurity and fear. look tough, act important.
5. deceptive 2 charming/manipulative	hide your true intentions. charm others, use them to get what you need.
6. burdened/enduring	bear up and wait it out.
7. expressive/clinging	dramatize events and feelings to get attention and avoid separation.
8. industrious/ over focused	work hard, keep going, let nothing distract you. take refuge in action.

Sensitive-Withdrawn. A person in a sensitive-withdrawn pattern uses the strategy of minimizing self-expression and emotional contact with self and others. The pattern reflects threats to survival and the core material will organize perceptions, feelings and actions around a theme of inescapable danger. On the surface, the basic uncertainty will be about whether or not one is welcome or belongs here. Feeling like strangers in a strange and dangerous land, these people strongly limit self-expression and contact with others. When the pattern is deeply ingrained, some of the following traits show up consistently: the person is withdrawn, shy, prefers isolation, especially under stress; likes to analyze, think, theorize, fantasize, imagine; they may seem cold, without emotions, unfriendly; Dr. Spock, though fictional, is a good example; the person's movements may be stiff and/or awkward, bodies are often thin and very tense and tight[6].

Dependent-Endearing. A person in a dependent-endearing pattern uses the strategy of seeking support by acting childlike and in need. The pattern reflects a lack of reliable nourishment and the core material will organize perceptions, feelings and actions around themes of poverty, loneliness, abandonment and loss. On the surface, the basic uncertainty will be about whether or not one will ever find reliable support. The person may feel there is some tragic flaw in them that makes them unacceptable to others and there is likely to be an inner rage about being abandoned. When the pattern is deeply ingrained, some of the following traits show up consistently: the person tends to give up easily; seeks help often but uses it poorly; has very low expectations, minimizes needs and wants and becomes depressed. In overall posture, they tend to collapse and have thin, soft, low tension bodies.

Self-reliant. A person in a self-reliant pattern uses the strategy of mobilizing self-support and proving self-reliance. The pattern reflects a decision to take care of oneself and not ever rely on others. The core material will organize perceptions, feelings and actions around themes of challenge and going it alone. Surface behavior will reflect these themes in activities of personal challenge, like mountain climbing, and in the simple fact of doing things for themselves without expecting help from anyone. Even in the therapy process, the person will seem to do all the work themselves. The culture figure is the cowboy, the lone gunfighter. When the pattern is deeply ingrained, some of the following traits show up consistently: the person seeks isolation under stress, likes to work alone, is active, takes on challenges, expects no help from others, has a slightly thin, strong body, with wide shoulders.

Deceptive I: Tough-Generous. A person in this pattern uses the strategy of giving the impression, one way or the other, that they are more intelligent, stronger, tougher, more important and/or more in charge than they really are. Often, they are also generous and take care of others. The pattern reflects a need to deceive and manipulate and the core material will organize perceptions, feelings and actions around themes of using others and being used by them. The person in this pattern is deeply invested in his or her personal image, in the impression he or she makes. On the surface, the basic uncertainty will be about whether or not one is respected and in control. The surface behavior will feel "slick" and elusive. The person usually has a desire to be in a position of power or authority — on top, the best, the leader. The person is willing to be supportive of others as long as he or she is taken seriously and is treated with respect and admiration. When the pattern is deeply ingrained, some of the following traits show up consistently: a tendency to secrecy, great difficulty in simply being real and honest with others, and with being vulnerable, showing hurt or weakness. The body tends to be large and blown up on top. The impression is one of exaggerated size. Culture heroes are: Superman, famous generals, football players, tough guys and exceptional talents. This type is also adventurous, creative and in the street version, criminal and antisocial.

Deceptive II: Charming-Manipulative. A person in this pattern uses the strategy of charming, tricking, seducing or manipulating others to get what he or she wants or needs. People using this strategy are similar to those in a tough-generous pattern. They are both deceptive, in this case about motives and their true feelings, in the other, about strength and power. Both types try to control others; one uses power and generosity, the other uses seduction and charm. The pattern reflects a need to hide who one really is. Core material will organize perceptions, feelings and actions around themes of being attractive, wanted, being exposed in some way, caught, found out, humiliated. On the surface, the basic uncertainty will be about whether or not one can have one's needs met in a straightforward way. The expectation is that others will use one's needs and vulnerabilities against one. Like the tough guys, this type feels insincere and phony. When the pattern is deeply ingrained, some of the following traits show up consistently: the person tries to make himself or herself attractive; movements are lithe and seductive, plus a lot of real charm and sweetness; often there are strong sexual overtones to their behavior and movements and a wider range of sexual activities than average; the body is supple and attractive.

Burdened-Enduring. A person in this pattern uses the strategy of bearing up (under the stress, strain, responsibility, obligations, pressure to change, move, grow up...) to delay and resist the other and wait it out. They use endurance to outlast troublesome situations and delay to avoid being controlled by others. People using this strategy take on the weight of events without making a serious effort to change things. Their strength is to endure. The pattern reflects issues of control and guilt. Attempts (and perceived attempts) to control the person are countered by delay and indirect defiance. "The harshest storms blow over soonest." The core material organizes perceptions, feelings and actions around themes of guilt, inadequacy, inferiority, of avoiding mistakes and hurting others, of being pushed and needing to resist, of being stuck and unable to express feelings. On the surface, the basic uncertainty will be about whether or not one can be effective, how well they can do things without making a mess of it and self-worth. This inhibits and delays action. When the pattern is deeply ingrained, some of the following traits show up consistently: the person feels stuck, impotent, incompetent and not as attractive or effective as other people. Under stress a person in this pattern will get stubborn, slow down, prepare for the worst and delay the inevitable. Being unbelievably patient, working years in the same dull job without promotion, the person acts and expects to be treated as "inferior" to others. The body tends to be short and thick, the kind that will hold up well under pressure. The person avoids responsibility and does not volunteer. He or she is quiet, a pillar of strength for others and may choose the role of martyr. At the same time, the person will tend to admire those outgoing, light, adventurous people so different from themselves.

Expressive-Clinging. A person in this pattern uses the strategy of dramatizing events and feelings to get and keep attention and to avoid separation. People who use this strategy are excitable and demonstrative; they get and keep others involved. The pattern reflects unfulfilled needs for attention and affection and difficulty accepting that one can be looked at and listened to without the drama. The core material will organize perceptions, feelings and actions around themes of separation and being pushed away and being loved, cared for, appreciated and attended to. On the surface, the basic uncertainty will be about whether or not one is interesting, attractive or wanted. When the pattern is deeply ingrained, some of the following traits show up consistently: the person is easily upset and often makes a show of it. He or she can be loud and/or very emotional. The person can be very caring, motherly, especially as part of an ongoing relationship. Or the person can be seductive, in a flamboyant, attention-getting way, or girlish and innocent, if that will keep things going. People in this pattern delay separations of all kinds and have trouble completing a conversation or a relationship. They can feel anxious or very sensitive. Their ability to dramatize is aided by an ability to amplify small feelings or sensations, making them extremely sensitive when they want to be. Many people with psychic abilities are in this pattern. The body tends, especially in women to be full and sexually attractive.

Industrious/Over focused. A person in this pattern uses the strategy of working hard, persisting and resisting distractions. The person takes refuge in action. The pattern reflects a need for achievement and recognition. The core material will organize perceptions, feelings and actions around themes of perfection, competition, failure, effort and striving and not being loved for oneself. On the surface, the basic uncertainty will be about whether or not one is worthy in the eyes of significant others, whether one is competent, adult and successful. When the pattern is deeply ingrained, some of the following traits show up consistently: people with this strategy are workaholic and serious, interested primarily in getting the job done right and then doing the next job even better. The person feels unappreciated and under pressure to perform. Like the expressive-clinging type, they have difficulties completing jobs and relationships. They are quick to feel frustration and anger. They make wonderful breadwinners, are perfectionistic, may seem cold to others and business like. Under stress they generate more effort and work even harder. They love action and doing and have strong, often athletic, bodies. Their heroes are the great achievers.

The Experience That Wants to Happen

In the course of growth, certain natural functions emerge, such as standing, walking, talking, and so on. We can look at character patterns as interruptions of, or impairments in, the growth of these natural psychological and social functions.

Impairment leaves the function truncated, distorted or incompletely learned. Without the successful learning of these functions, certain experiences never get to happen. The goal of therapy is to create and integrate those experiences, which in the normal course of growth, should have happened, but didn't. What follows is a list of the missing core experiences for each character pattern.

1. sensitive-withdrawn	safety, being welcome, being here in the world, pleasurable contact... freedom from terror
2. dependent-endearing	gratitude, being cared for, abundance, bonded, nourished... freedom from want
3. self-reliant	willing support from others... freedom from challenge
4. tough-generous	being real, showing weakness, needs... freedom from being used, manipulated
5. charming-manipulative	being real, acceptance of self as it really is... freedom from persecution
6. burdened-enduring	absence of pressure, responsibility, guilt, freedom to do for self, to express
7. expressive-clinging	freely given love and attention, not to have to struggle for attention, freedom to rely on relationships
8. industrious-overfocused	to be loved, appreciated, just for who you are, freedom to relax and play

Character Basics

Basics, like nervous system function, biological adaptation, development, social interaction and experiential organization do not "explain" character in the reductionistic sense. They simply provide points of view which can be used to think about the individuals we work with. People's structure and behavior offer clues to their core material only to the extent that we have viewpoints from which to perceive and understand. By including this small section, I mean to suggest that it is worth our while to relate character to wider fields, especially to biology and to systems theory.

Some Underlying Dimensions of Character

I have chosen a few dimensions which have proved of value. I borrowed these dimensions from Milton Erickson, Carl Jung and David Shapiro[7]. They represent a current area of interest and study in psychology, and a good deal of literature on the subject can be found.

Milton K. Erickson's Dimensions

1. Attention	internal/external
	focused/diffuse
2. Distance	absorbed/objective
3. Suggestion	direct/indirect
4. Control	one-up/one-down/equal

David Shapiro's Dimensions

1. Focus	open/narrow
2. Thinking	global/detailed
3. Actions	impulsive/inhibited

Jung's Dimensions

The Types	thinking/feeling/sensing/intuiting
	introvert/extrovert

Hakomi Dimensions

1. Dispositions	withdraw/collapse/deceive
	resist/dramatize/action
2. Cortical Control	inhibited/impulsive
3. ANS	sympathetic/parasympathetic

Discussion

Attention: is an input function. It involves operations that modify and control the flow of information into the system. It deals largely with how the world is perceived and the beginnings of any attempt to deal with the world. Attention functions are especially important in any information overload situation. The dimensions of attention are: internal/external and focused or diffuse.

Internal/external. For any individual, at a particular time, the focus of attention will be either on external events (using the distance receptors) or on internal events (sensing body position, feelings, hunger, internal temperature, etc.) Of course one can attend to both at once, or one can alternate rapidly from internal to external. Some people have the flexibility of attention to do such things. What is significant for the study of character is the fixation at or strong preference for one locus of attention over another. (This is true for every dimension. Character patterns are limitations even at the level of these underlying variables.)

Those who attend internally have slight delays in their responses as they take in the world and convert it to inner experience. They will have less trouble knowing their feelings and other internal events and possibly more trouble dealing with others, new places, new people, crowds, noise and such. This way of attending relates to Jung's introverted type. External attenders are more directly coupled to the world around them and have some difficulty knowing their own internal states. They are related to Jung's extraverted type and are more comfortable with other people than are internal attenders.

We see this dimension operating in the expressive and industrious patterns. For example, the expressives have a more internal attention and the industrious, external. The ease with which expressives (people in dependent-endearing patterns, too) can report feelings is one sign of internal attention. Mindfulness, of course, is training for internal attention.

Focused/diffuse. Attention can be narrowly or widely focused. It can be open to new inputs from new sources, taking in wide areas of interest and staying flexible towards whatever enters. Or it can be narrowed and pointed, staying with one thing and not allowing new inputs or interruptions. It can be oriented towards overall patterns or rooted in details. And, as with all the dimensions, it can be flexible and capable of going from one form to another. For those with more open focus, larger, more global areas are covered and can be integrated, but detail is lost. The narrow focus has the complementary qualities of picking up the fine details and losing the overall picture. Shapiro's dimension of focus, narrow or diffuse, is the same as that of Erickson's attention dimension, focused or diffuse. It is worth noting that more than one thinker in this field has come up with the same handful of variables.

This variable is closely related to control issues and thinking styles. It takes a high degree of control to maintain focus in the face of large disturbance. I remember a photograph of Nikola Tesla sitting in his laboratory with the largest and most elaborate discharges of electricity going on around him, like a vast electric storm above his head, while he sat quietly reading a book. It was a joke, of course. Yet there are those who can calmly attend to an image of God while their very bodies burn, as we saw in Vietnam. It takes a narrow focus of attention, as David Shapiro has pointed out, to support a style of thinking like the paranoid style. Diffuse focus is more characteristic of the person with an expressive-clinging style, who experiences a sense of the whole scene and the general feeling of the situation rather than details. The thinking style of the expressive is global also, more general, more people and pattern-oriented, cooking by taste and intuition, without the use of recipes and measuring spoons.

Distance. We can be totally absorbed, oblivious to everything else, losing the sense of time, place and even self. To be so absorbed is to close the distance between oneself and whatever one is attending to. Or we can feel separate, not involved, as if everything were going on at a great distance, behind a glass wall, out of our personal field and in no way involving the self. In the extreme, this is the ideal of objectivity and objective science. It is about whether we throw ourselves wholeheartedly into our interactions or stay at a distance.

Absorption. Relates to the strong social needs and propensities of the parasympathetic types. Their involvement with others and their biases around nourishment and nurturing all require absorption. The distancers, like the sensitive-withdrawn pattern people and others with high sympathetic nervous system activity, are more able to keep to themselves and to look with cool eyes at those around them.

Thinking Style. Thinking, like focus, can be global or detailed. The fine-grained, analytic style of thinking tends to lose the practical, broad meaning of things. At its most narrow it is the thinking of the paranoid looking for clues while the true fabric of the immediate situation is pushed out of focus. The global, impressionistic style of thinking has the true feel of events and is often thought of as intuitive. It is the particulars which are thought of as unimportant and so are lost. This dimension is important to the therapist since it is necessary in the course of therapy to move from one style to the other.

The expressive-clinging style is more global, the sensitive-withdrawn and the industrious, more narrow. In therapy, one person will describe very detailed reactions to a probe, reporting, say, a singular sensation like a tingling in one finger, while another will report a total bodily feeling. Their thinking will also be different along the same lines. This is one of Shapiro's dimensions and he covers it in great detail in his books[8].

Action. Actions are somewhere along a dimension which goes from the highly controlled, planned and premeditated, circumscribed and deliberate to the opposite extreme of completely spontaneous, unplanned, spur-of-the-moment, unexpected and impulsive. The burdened-enduring is over controlled in the extreme whereas the expressive-clinging is often unrestrained.

Suggestion. This refers to whether a person will respond to direct or indirect suggestion. It has a lot to do with sensitivity to being manipulated or treated roughly. The parasympathetics, with their fine social sense and tact, are more likely to respond to indirect suggestions and the more sympathetic to direct ones.

Control. This has to do with where one likes to put oneself or find oneself in relationships. Some people prefer the security and shared responsibility of the equals position. They want to be treated as equals and will resist any attempt either to put them in charge or to subordinate them. A multiple channels strategy might use a control position like this. Others prefer to be one-up or one-down. The one-downers, like the burdened-enduring and the dependent-endearing, seek to have the other take responsibility. The one-uppers are willing to do that for whatever privileges accrue to the position. It is for this reason that you'll often find people in dependent-endearing patterns or burdened pattern people in close relationships with people in tough-generous patterns.

Jung's typology gives us introverts, extroverts, feeling types, and so on. Dr. Edward Wilson of Colorado University[9] relates these types to physiological variables such as brain wave frequencies, neuro-transmitters and preferred stress paths. According to Wilson, the different Jungian types have preferences about where they put their stress — into the muscular, cardiovascular, neuronal or endocrine systems. The sensing types put their stress mostly in the muscular system, the feeling types, in the endocrine or hormonal system. The thinking types prefer cardiovascular involvement and the intuitives use neuronal stress paths. Dr. Wilson is still experimenting and as far as I know, hasn't published his findings yet. In Hakomi, the character patterns each include a particular disposition. These dispositions are biases toward the end points of what should be balanced continuums. Further information on character patterns is given in Chapter 17, Barriers and Character.

The field of character theory is an old and extensive one. I would like to recommend particularly the books of: Steven Johnson, Alexander Lowen, John Pierrakos, Wilhelm Reich and David Shapiro. For a systems theory perspective, see the book, *Family Evaluation* by Michael Kerr and Murry Bowen, W.W. Norton & Company, New York, 1988.

Notes for Chapter 3.

1. All the Chinese are different from each other, as are Whites and Blacks and Native American people. Yet, we can all tell a Chinese from a Black, a Black from a White, etc. Character patterns are not a denial of uniqueness, just a limitation on it.

2. See James Miller's seminal work, Living Systems. New York: McGraw-Hill Book Co., 1977. Miller describes eight adjustment processes to information overload: omissions, errors, filtering, abstracting, multiple channels, queuing, escape and chunking. Some of the connections of overload adjustment and character strategies are given in the section on character as strategy.

3. For a fine treatment of personal mythology, see David Feinstein and Stanley Kripner's, Personal Mythology: The Psychology of Your Evolving Self. Los Angeles: Jeremy P. Tarcher, Inc., 1988.

4. Alexander Lowen, Narcissism: The Denial of the True Self. New York: MacMillan, 1983.

5. For a long time, I used the names for character types given by Freud, Reich and Lowen. The correspondences are as follows: sensitive-withdrawn was schizoid; dependent-endearing, oral; self-reliant, compensated oral; deceptive one and two, psychopath; burdened-enduring, masochist; expressive-clinging, hysteric; industrious-overfocused, phallic. It seemed time to drop these clinical, disease-oriented classifications.

6. For a discussion of how the body reflects each of these character patterns, see both The Body Reveals by Kurtz and Prestera, New York: Harper & Row, Publishers, 1976 and Ken Dychtwald's Bodymind, New York: Jove Publications, Inc. 1978.

7. See David Shapiro's, Neurotic Styles, New York: Basic Books, Inc. 1965 and Autonomy and Rigid Character, New York: Basic Books, Inc. 1981; and Milton Erickson and Ernest and Sheila Rossi's, Hypnotic Realities, New York: Irvington Publishers, Inc., 1976; and Anthony Storr's, The Essential Jung, Princeton, New Jersey: Princeton University Press, 1983.

8. ibid.

9. Personal communication.

4

HEALING RELATIONSHIP

*The basic work of health professionals in general, and of
psychotherapists in particular, is to become full human beings
and to inspire full human-beingness in other people who feel
starved about their lives.*

- Chogyam Trungpa, Becoming A Full Human Being

The best leader follows.

- Lao Tzu, Tao Te Ching

---

*All real living is meeting. Meeting is not in time and space,
but space and time in meeting.*

- Martin Buber

Introduction: A Hierarchy of Contexts

In the development of Hakomi, a hierarchy of contexts emerged where each
new level served to inform and regulate the levels below. The level of technique
is the lowest. Techniques are tangible and easy to learn. You can learn to deliver
a probe in twenty minutes or so. (You won't learn all about probes in twenty
minutes, but you can learn to deliver them.) The techniques are very powerful and
they work. Students have some immediate success using them and the work is

very exciting at this point. Depending on their capacities and interests, students may work at this level for months or, sometimes, years. There is a lot of technique to learn. While learning is still centered on this level, the techniques tend to be overused. In the early stages, students are taking over everything in sight and doing probes at a terrifying rate. The student still fascinated with technique uses a frame of mind that demands an awareness of small details. In that frame of mind, the student is not yet able to sense the larger contexts. The student is searching for opportunities to use the techniques he or she has learned and doesn't yet know much about actively creating those opportunities. With experience, more and more such opportunities are noticed and gradually the problem becomes which ones to chose. Finally, the question of why one technique and not another emerges. So, a combination of mastery and frustration finally motivates a shift in focus, away from techniques themselves to a way to organize the use of techniques in an integrated, systematic fashion. Technique has become habit. The next level emerges: method.

The method, as the next higher level, organizes the use of the techniques. In studying the method, one begins to think about: what character process is this? What system am I in and how can I jump out? What part of the process is this? How do I create an experiment here? How can I get some more information about this or that? Is this a good time to do a little experiment? What shall I contact? All those are questions about method and process and character. One becomes powerfully aware of the larger aspects of the client as a whole person. For example, the student learns to recognize, contact and work with the child part of the client. This is exciting and the work feels somehow new. At this level, the student learns to do more with less. He uses the techniques less, with more precision. The student also learns character patterns and strategies and uses them in the work. The student begins to step back from the moment to moment details to notice larger patterns. These larger patterns: managing consciousness, lowering the noise, establishing mindfulness, gathering information, evoking experiences, studying the organization of experience, working with emotional release, the child, transformation, integration, and so forth, are the concerns of the method.

It takes much longer to master this level. There's a lot to learn and it must be assimilated, made habit. A long time must be spent studying and practicing. The work becomes a full-time preoccupation. At this level the work also comes truly alive. It becomes richer and more satisfying. The student works more confidently with a wider variety of people on ever deeper levels. The method can help one become a powerful therapist. Still, even the method has it's limits.

After a long time and much practice, we come to feel limited again. The method isn't enough somehow. So, we look for a larger context, something beyond the method, just as method is beyond technique. This is the level of relationship. The method is embedded in the context of the therapist-client relationship. It is this relationship that determines when methods work and when they don't. At this level, the therapist's emotional growth and depth of understanding are crucial. Here we begin to use our full selves, our human-beingness. There is still much at this level that the student needs to learn.

As my understanding went from one level to another, my ability to do therapy increased dramatically. It seems that when a new level is needed, understanding gathers momentum until, rather suddenly, a new organizing principle becomes clear. After I had accumulated so much detail about the method that it became conceptually unwieldy, something quite simple emerged to organize it. What emerged was a vision in which the building of a special relationship with the client takes precedence over all else. This essence of this relationship is the cooperation of the unconscious. It depends upon two complex structures: the emotional attitude of the therapist and the therapist's understanding of the client's world.

The principles are the highest level of context. The principles guide all levels of development, but especially our capacity for a healing relationship. The emotional attitude of the therapist is grounded in the principles. When I work with advanced students, it is this that we work with. We focus on how each of us still has work to do on ourselves, how each of us can still learn more about how to "rest within the principles." To rest within unity, we have to learn that healing is not a function of the therapist or any external agent like a vitamin or an antibiotic. Healing and control are with the client and are functions of the client-therapist relationship. Knowing that, knowing I don't control the process, I avoid efforting. And knowing the client also cannot force change at a deep level, I encourage the client to drop efforting.

I was leading a workshop. The group was split into small groups of four or five, doing an exercise that often evokes strong emotions and processing. When things were well under way, I walked around and came to a woman working with expressions of resistance. She was lying down with several people gently restraining her arms and legs. She was pushing her arms and legs against the resistance of the others and pushing out some expressions of, "No! I won't. You can't treat me this way." Things like that. Another group member, a therapist of a more aggressive persuasion, was directing. She was holding the struggler's arms at the wrists. With each movement or spoken expression, the therapist would say, "Good! Good!" As soon as I saw this, I wasn't happy. I didn't know exactly why but, for me, something was wrong.

I sat down beside this little group and looked at the therapist. I told her that I would like to take over at this point and I invited her to watch my approach. She was agreeable. I didn't know what I was going to do; I only knew I didn't like what was going on. As I've thought about it since, I realize I didn't like the efforting. I didn't like the sense I got of the client working at expression, pushing for it, struggling. I didn't like seeing the therapist controlling the process and encouraging the efforting. I like to see the spontaneous happening.

Effort is an ego function. When one efforts, the act of efforting creates an I and a something the I struggles against. In this drama of struggle and competition, the chief act is the creation of a separate self: an ego. Without the struggle there is no drama and no dramatis personae. With the spontaneous, effort evaporates and ego relaxes. This relaxation is essential for healing. This relaxation is not a passive giving up, but a giving in to the process, a faith in something deeper in oneself, in realms beyond the ego. In Hakomi, we work deliberately for the support of the larger selves of both therapist and client. Our way of working recognizes healing as something very different from anything the therapist or even the limited conscious ego of the client can do. Our present cultural and personal myths are too much a celebration of the ego. Our notions of separate self are out of balance with all sorts of larger selves: family, community, the biological world, the universe and God. All too easily, we feel ourselves to be separate from these larger selves. In our imagined isolation, not knowing the help we could get, we struggle.

So, I asked the "client" to slow down and relax for a moment. With a little reluctance, she did that. I asked her to go inside and find, "what wants to happen." What movement wants to happen? What expression? What resistance from those holding her would feel exactly right. This one question shifts the locus of control from the therapist to some unnamed intelligence inside the client. I didn't ask her what she wants, just what wants. By doing that, I'm really asking her to contact some larger self within. I'm asking for a relaxation of effort, for a turning inward and for increased awareness. This shift to relaxation and awareness is a big part of resting in the principles and creating a healing relationship.

She began to adjust. She felt better with the legs and arms going more slowly. We slowed down to support her process. She became clearer and clearer that, at the level of what wants to happen, these movements were the right ones. They felt good. At that point, I encouraged her to stay with them as long as they felt that way and to wait for anything else that wanted to happen. After getting the feeling right, I imagined that the next step might be curiosity. I thought she might begin wondering, "why do these particular movements feel so good?" So, I was just sitting there and she was having a very pleasant time, playing you might say. Her expressions seemed to have a quality of delicious and righteous rebellion. I wasn't directing her movements or even encouraging one over another. I had simply directed a shift from the external reinforcements of the therapist to the internal authority of her own feelings.

Sure enough, she started to get curious. It happened quite spontaneously. Curiosity is a powerful tool and a great ally in therapy[1]. We all want to understand. The significant thing here is that the experience came first, then the need for understanding emerged. We must wait to search for understanding until the client is experiencing a present experience that he or she is naturally curious about. To engage any other way tends more to substitute for feelings than to make sense of them. So, in Hakomi, we establish present experience as our focus, support feelings and expression and only then go for meaning. So, when her curiosity emerged, I asked some questions about the meaning of her experience: "what type of movements are these? What is your body saying with these movements? What words go with this experience?" I told her, "don't try to think of words! Let the words come from some place within you! You just listen for them!" Again, I ask for no effort and the support of the larger field. I invite the unconscious to participate.

Well, quite suddenly she remembered: they had never allowed her to crawl. Those movements looked exactly like crawling. It all made sense now. It was about her right to move her own body the way she wanted. From that point on I worked with helping her take in the knowledge that she didn't always have to fight for her freedom. I told her it was okay to crawl, that no one would interfere. Someone might even help. She could get support for what she wanted and needed. She wouldn't always be fighting bigger, stronger people — and losing. That felt good. She took it in and felt relief. She relaxed more and got more memories and insights. The whole process turned out well. In the end, she felt wonderful. She understood a lot about where her battle for freedom had come from and she could see herself dropping that whole drama. Freedom was now, simply hers to own.

If you followed the broad flow of the process here, you will have gathered that it starts with helping the person relax and turn inward towards present experience, establishing and supporting mindfulness. The fundamental activity here is self study, with less doing, and more just being and following. Then, we make ready for, contact, evoke, welcome and nurture some naturally unfolding growth process. When such processes happen spontaneously, it is a clear sign that the unconscious is cooperating, that the larger self is participating. This backing off and letting things happen is essential for healing and the cooperation of the unconscious. It is a cardinal example of nonviolence at its most effective. The connection to the creation of a healing relationship here is that I invited the unconscious and got its cooperation.

The Cooperation of The Unconscious

The goal and primary result of establishing a successful relationship is the cooperation of the client at an unconscious level. The client slips into an easy, working relationship, with no need to resist. The therapist has established herself or himself as non-threatening and understanding of the client's experiences.

Without the cooperation of the unconscious, the therapy process moves very slowly, if at all. The method doesn't work. The client very automatically and unconsciously slows down or deflects the process. When the client resists, it is justified resistance. If the therapist is not being sensitive to something the client needs, something about safety or being understood, then the client will resist. It is a mistake to attempt to work at the level of method before the relationship is firmly established.

The unconscious has great power to make things happen. When the therapist has the cooperation of the unconscious, the process moves along smoothly, without effort. The therapist can use technique and method much more sparingly. The establishment of relationship and cooperation is prior to the method and it is what makes the method effective. The maintenance of the relationship takes precedence over anything else that's happening within the process, except for staying within the principles. When the client is giving signals that indicate that the unconscious is beginning to resist, it is wise to back off whatever you are doing and start thinking about and working on the relationship again.

Basic to the cooperation of the unconscious is the ability to relate to it directly. This involves a couple of things. One is reading the signs which tell about unconscious beliefs, attitudes and present experience. The other is the ability to respond to those signs appropriately. These skills are usually learned over several years. They depend heavily upon two aspects of the therapist which mature over time: (1) the therapist's understanding, experience and wisdom and (2) the therapist's emotional attitude.

The unconscious speaks through mood, feeling, posture, tone of voice, pace, facial expression. Here are short lists of some of the signs of cooperation and how the therapist earns it, and of resistance and how the therapist evokes it:

Signs of Cooperation and How It Is Earned:

1. The client offers thoughtful answers to the therapist's questions; earned by: asking questions that are useful, of immediate interest to the client (rather than just the therapist), questions that are not just ways to hide or keep busy...
2. Attention to and consideration of the therapist's statement earned by: the same consideration and attention given to the client, shown by understanding not just the words, but the attitudes and feelings present...
3. A concentrated attention to the present interaction; earned by: attention to the present, ability to stay with the present even when the client drifts off into memories, speculation or generalizations...
4. Interactions that reflect inclusion of the therapist in the client's process; earned by: an awareness of that process and a willingness to give priority to the client's needs and direction, that is, to drop one's own agenda in favor of the client's when this is evoking resistance...
5. The client goes along with the therapist's suggestions; earned by: the ability to judge when and how to take charge and the resources to make good use of being in charge...

6. Concentration and a general willingness to participate; earned by: understanding and resting in the principles...

Signs of Resistance and How It Is Evoked by the Therapist:

1. The client slows the process down, not answering questions, not taking suggestions seriously; evoked by: misreading the signs, not giving the client the time he or she needs to just think, pushing for ones own agenda rather than discovering the client's...

2. The client takes off on his or her own directions without connecting with the therapist first; evoked by: not taking charge at the appropriate times; not being clear about what the client is experiencing when he or she is unhappy with the way things are going; not jumping out of the system soon enough...

3. Yawns, distractions, delays, arguments, intellectual discussions, speaking in a casual way; evoked by: not addressing the real concerns of the client...

Good therapy has a feel to it. It feels easy and right. There's movement from superficial concerns to deeper levels of interest, curiosity, feeling and insight. There is also spontaneity. New, surprising things happen. There are discoveries. There are times of being stuck, times of fear and despair, but the general feeling is one of movement, progress. All the signs of unconscious cooperation are there. When the unconscious cooperates, significant material emerges. In a good session, client and therapist both participate fully, each allowing the other an important place in the work. The flavor is one of mutuality and significance. Feelings arise and are expressed. The client relives and resolves painful memories. Old patterns are made conscious and new patterns are explored. The motive forces which energize and direct these changes originate within the client. The motive forces are growth processes which have had a difficult time maturing. Something has been interrupting them, some once powerful need to act against one's own growth. Whatever it is, it frustrated growth and development, first, in the normal growth periods of childhood, and later, as part of an adapted, general approach to life. The potential for growth is there waiting. Good therapy recognizes it.

The Emotional Attitude of the Therapist: Resting in Nonviolence

Even more important, good therapy avoids triggering the need to resist. For that, a warm, accepting emotional attitude is essential, especially accepting of the defenses and strong needs for safety and control that the defenses represent. Those needs are mostly unconscious and so, are extremely potent. No matter what difficulties and pain they cause the client, within the client's present belief system, they are logical and necessary. Acknowledging the defenses and honoring them, allows them to relax and makes way for important experiences to emerge. In working with defenses, we recognize, acknowledge and accept them, without judgment. Any other emotional attitude evokes them and entangles the therapist in the client's conflicts and character systems. Acceptance without judgment is crucial and it is not easy. It requires a deep understanding of oneself as well as the client. It must be part of the emotional makeup of the therapist, not something one simulates as part of one's role. The unconscious will not be fooled by simulations. It has to be real. Such a mature emotional attitude allows the therapist to step back easily from his or her own agendas[2]. An effortless yielding of one's agendas is a major signal to the client's unconscious that here is a person I do not have to resist.

Often the client's usual way of being in an intimate relationship also interferes with the smooth operations of the method. The client may not contact feelings easily. The client may not like instructions or normally volunteer information or initiate interactions. The client may ask many questions or always try to please. There are many such patterns. They derive from the rules for living in certain families and may be quite different from the rules the therapist grew up with. An openness to such diversity is crucial. To gain the cooperation of the unconscious, the therapist may have to let go of a need to be doing what he or she wants to do. That's not always easy. Our intentions and habits are not always conscious or controllable. We like to participate and feel effective. We want to do things to help the client. After all, therapy is our job and we like doing it.

But when we're into doing, the client is all too easily seen as part of our process, working for us, helping us to help them. With that attitude, we easily get frustrated and blame our frustrations on the client. We think of the client's defenses as something to be broken through and overcome. Or we just subtly, even unconsciously feel that. From the client's perspective, especially unconsciously, there is something in this attitude any healthy person would feel compelled to resist. At least a part of them wants to resist, even if there is some conscious agreement that it is all for the client's good. Subtle though it may be and based on the best intentions, it is still force. Even in the name of love, violence is violence and is inevitably resisted. Cooperation of the unconscious happens when the client finds nothing in the therapist to resist.

The immature therapist has trouble backing off. Frustration comes easily and is usually answered with more technique and method. Stepping back is letting go of doing things and just taking a look at what's going on. This taking in without immediately needing to do something is the beginning of wisdom and similar to mindfulness. It is the difference between reactions and responses. For example, the therapist doesn't speak every time the client speaks. The therapist waits a few moments before replying to the client. The therapist makes a simple contact statement about the essence of what the client presents and waits patiently to see what the client does with it. These are signs that the therapist is not lost in the details, not caught up in the system. This patience and openness are signals to the client's unconscious that the therapist is not there to impose anything, to force anything. They are signs that the therapist is alert and sensitive to the needs of client and has the right emotional attitude. From the therapists point of view it means creating an ever expanding ability to accept who the client is at any moment. The right emotional attitude allows the therapist to be ready to help and just as ready to back off and wait. The therapist must be able to reverse at any moment, to back off and wait, to step back and grasp the connections from a larger perspective.

A mature attitude also allows the therapist to use what's wrong with a session, when something is keeping the process shallow and unproductive, when the process feels strained and uncertain and the connection isn't right. Nothing's happening. Feelings like these are signals. They tell the therapist to slow down, step back and focus on what's wrong. They may not be spoken of with the client necessarily, but they must be consciously, deliberately thought about. For experienced therapists, this is done habitually. Frustration, discontent, boredom, confusion, these are signals. They tell the therapist to look for something systematic going on with the client or between the client and oneself[3].

For the client, defense systems are habits which manage the flow of experience. Sensing and studying them is a way to avoid being stopped by them. If we notice them and act quickly, the process doesn't bog down, but gains the added momentum of a natural interest in present feelings and relationships. They may also clarify one's own emotional needs or bring some understanding of the client's world. With too much drive to make something happen and too much attachment to the method, the therapist's tendency will be to ignore such signals, to push them out of consciousness in order to get on with the business of therapy. But they are the business of therapy and the better we use them, the better therapy will go.

Here's a little story about signals: every morning, a worker crossed the border on a bicycle. A guard suspected that the worker was smuggling something. The guard searched the worker every time he crossed, without ever finding anything. Still, the guard was right. The man was a smuggler. He was smuggling bicycles. If therapy is to go well, we must detect and respond to signals that tell us something is wrong. We're all smugglers. We all bring our character patterns into therapy in the guise of everyday things. Listen to the signals that tell you that. Don't push them out of your mind just to get on with therapy. If you sense something is wrong, focus on that sense, understand where it's coming from. Look into and take care of such things. By giving the relationship the higher priority, the use of method and technique actually becomes easier. Once the cooperation of the unconscious is gained, the process unfolds smoothly, with little effort. The same deep needs that inform character and defense, inform the client-therapist relationship. Therapy begins here, because it must.

The Cooperation of One's Own Unconscious: Intuitive Body Reading, An Example

A healing relationship also requires that the therapist have the cooperation of his or her own unconscious, in order to be creative and intuitive. Learning to read bodies for psychological information is a good example of relating to your own unconscious. There are two very different approaches to body reading and they reflect two different ways of operating in the world, two different paradigms. One way attempts to be objective and relies on theory, logic and memory. The other includes feelings and personal experience and relies on intuition and direct knowing. When I first learned body reading, I learned both ways. The first was about what each body part can tell us. I learned that mostly by reading Alexander Lowen's books. I learned by reading about what the body meant, part by part. This approach is understanding through special knowledge. An authority with special knowledge imparts to others through books, lectures, and examples. This way is left brained and rational and feels like taking something in from the outside.

That's the first way I learned. I learned that body structure, posture, and the various parts and features all have meaning. I just learned those meanings and practiced looking at people with those meanings in mind. It seemed that I needed nothing more. Just memorize the list and understand the reasons for each part meaning what it does and you can read bodies. It was very analytical, fixed and linear. There was nothing about the unconscious or the observer, nothing about states of consciousness or feelings. It's a list of what means what. In theory, anyone could learn it and use it. It wasn't about intentions or relationships or special talents.

I learned a second way to read bodies by studying a little while directly with John Pierrakos. Pierrakos is famous for reading bodies (auras, too). I made photographic slides of my clients and brought them to John. We sat together, I'd show a slide and he'd comment. He'd say things like, "the pools of stagnation." This wasn't from any list that I knew of. This was John's unconscious speaking. He would open to and resonate with the person on the screen. The person's deepest issues and emotional history spoke to John. I knew these people. I knew them from long hours in therapy. I knew that something in John, something intuitive, was connecting. That was his way. Just watching him, I learned. He taught me that there was more to knowing than parts from a list. He had learned to see people directly. He could have made a parts list anytime he wanted. He didn't need one.

John's work wasn't about special knowledge but rather about a special connection to his own unconscious gifts. He had developed something there inside him. We can each develop our own gifts. To do so, we must connect with parts of our minds we are not usually conscious of. We have to learn a whole new way to be with ourselves. This new way invites the participation of the unconscious. It involves a different way of learning and it creates different skills. Body reading is only a very minor one. A cultivated, inner wisdom must inform the work. That wisdom tells you how fast or slow to go, when to speak, and when to remain silent. It guides the healing process. It builds not just skills, but a healthy, loving way of being.

A few more words about connecting to your own unconscious: how is it that John Pierrakos can do these things and you can't? Why is this natural ability not operative for you, right now? Is it something that you failed to develop, or something the parenting figures talked you out of? Was there something wrong with it? When I explore these issues with students, we find cultural and family taboos about genuinely knowing, seeing and being with each other. There are family styles which discourage intuition and direct connections. There is a cultural bias which leads us to neglect and subvert our intuitive talents. Perhaps you once knew how and you put it aside, accepting the taboos against it and the general suspicions and low opinions of it. Perhaps you learned a whole other way of doing things, an active, physical way, full of competition and effort and clever argument. Or maybe, without much support, you just didn't know how.

In trying to connect with themselves and others, most people simply try too hard. If they have a little trouble at first, they become confused and frustrated and they begin to effort and struggle. They seem to be saying to themselves, "I should be able to do this. If I just try hard enough, I will be able to do it." It's as if they were lifting weights. It's as if minds had no reality or influence and all reality was ponderous material. Instead of relaxing and waiting, seeing where the process wants to go, they take charge and try to steer the process too strongly. The client's unconscious is very likely to be sensitive to that. Most people have worked hard for whatever freedom and autonomy they enjoy. They balk when someone challenges or threatens them. If the therapist tries too hard, too long, something in them quits or never shows up. Client and therapist may continue, they may go through the motions of being in therapy, but is no more than an empty ritual. Unconsciously, cooperation has ceased.

The same will happen if you try to force your own unconscious. When you're not curious any more, just working, when the work isn't playful and spontaneous, it won't be creative. The unconscious will stop participating. When you feel playful and open and fresh, when you put aside the struggle to be right or in charge, when you embrace the process as a gift, gratefully, willing to learn from it, okay that it isn't all explainable, when you are willing to begin simply, with what is there in the client and in yourself, when you are available to the full range of experience, joy, pain, fear, courage, love, hate, all this, then it will be easy. Then it will be full of surprises and delight and heartfelt moments.

When the Client Knows that the Therapist Understands:

Understanding is the other essential ingredient needed to gain the cooperation of the unconscious. The unconscious appreciates it when the therapist knows what's going on. If the therapist can show that he or she understands the immediate situation, the client's present experience, and can make intelligent conclusions about the client's past, something in the client will relax and allow the process to unfold further. It is very much like an ordinary conversation, only it is played out as process. The client needs to know that the therapist has understood the first thing before going on to the second. If the client is feeling sadness, the first thing that will help that sadness to deepen and progress will be some sign from the therapist that he or she is aware of it. Just a phrase, like, "Some sadness, huh," can be enough. This ability to understand (and to quietly demonstrate that you understand) is combined with a warm, accepting attitude, is the beginning of therapy.

In its full ripeness this understanding is the wisdom that comes from living your life fully, from years of deep interest in people, how they get to be who they are and what changes them. It comes from a passion for the truth about ourselves and others. In the language of systems theory, it comes from a large, well integrated, easily accessed data base. You must know a lot about people and have that knowing put together and ready to use. As in most effective systems, understanding and the right emotional attitude are mutually supportive; each sustains and enhances the other. To create cooperation, it takes both. And effort is no substitute.

A healing relationship is special. When you are in one, you feel it. There is an incredible delicacy that you do not dare to disturb. There is a connection with yourself that allows you to relax, be curious and wait. There are intuitions that pop up easily and make powerful contributions to the work. There is a basic warmth and friendliness. There's a basic wakefulness that informs both therapist and client. There is no question of healer and healed. Both are parts of something greater taking place. Both feel this. Each is healed.

Notes for Chapter 4.

1. See Gregory Johanson's, *A Curious Form of Therapy: Hakomi*, form the Hakomi Forum, issue no. 6, published in Boulder, CO., by the Hakomi Institute. Another nice article about this is, *Hypothesizing, Circularity, and Neutrality Revisited: An Invitation to Curiosity*, by Gianfranco Cecchin, M.D., Family Process, Vol 26, No. 4, December, 1987.

2. In *The Potent Self*, Moshe Feldenkrais describes a mature movement as one which can be reversed at any point. This ability to reverse or step back from one's actions signals maturity in a therapist also. There are four signs of mature movement: reversibility is one, effortlessness, lack of any sense of resistance, and unimpaired breathing are the others. They all apply as well to the therapists emotional attitude.

3. Much about this is covered in Chapter 17, Jumping Out of the System

SECTION TWO

THE PROCESS

Easy is right.
Begin right and
you are easy.

Continue easy and
you are right.

Chuang Tsu

5

THE ESSENTIAL PROCESS

An Expression of The Principles

Hakomi, as a method of psychotherapy, is unique because it is an expression of the principles. It is only one of many possible expressions. Other therapies use awareness. That is like using the mindful state, though awareness is not as specifically defined. Other therapies are humanistic and supportive and non-authoritarian. But none of that is nonviolence as we use it. It's close, but it is still within models that do not embrace the principles as a whole. It is this embracing of the principles which gives Hakomi real roots and grounding. The combined use of the principles as guidelines, mindfulness as a therapeutic tool, and nonviolence as a basic emotional attitude of the therapist make Hakomi unique. Ours is the method of evoked experiences in mindfulness. I don't know any other therapy that uses this particular method. The feeling is there. People come up to me after workshops and say they had an immediate affinity for the work. They had felt immediately that it was right for them, like they had been waiting for it. The rapport is there. I believe Hakomi simply expresses what many who teach or parent or do healing work already feel, but haven't found the exact words or precise method for.

The Method of Evoked Experiences in Mindfulness

The essential process is the frame for using the method of evoked experiences (Table 1). The process itself is framed by the healing relationship and that in turn by the principles. Within the frame of the process, we do three big things: we establish mindfulness; we evoke experiences of different kinds; and we process the experiences evoked in one of three different, state- specific ways. Let's look at the larger frames first. To establish mindfulness, a feeling of safety and an attitude of cooperation are needed. Safety is needed to relax "defenses" and to allow the open, vulnerable, sensitive state that mindfulness is. Cooperation is needed in order to be able to participate in the ongoing process. Cooperation is both conscious and unconscious; we especially want and work for the cooperation of the unconscious. It is gained by staying within the principles and by understanding the client. Once established, safety and cooperation set the stage for establishing and using mindfulness.

Figure 1. Evoked Experiences in Mindfulness

ESTABLISH MINDFULNESS	EVOKED EXPERIENCES		T*	STATE-SPECIFIC PROCESSING
M	feelings	images		
M M				
M M	thoughts	sensations		going for meaning
M M				
M M	tensions	impulses		strong emotions
M M				
M	memories	child		work with the child

*The letter T stands for the transition to processing. (Table 1)

Establishing Mindfulness

Mindfulness is a special state.[1] It is self-observing. It is noticing one's own present experience. It is also a special kind of availability, an openness of the mind, a willingness to allow oneself to be affected. Mindfulness is characterized by relaxed volition. It is a relaxed, open, undefended, quiet state. In mindfulness, one can be extremely sensitive. Small, precise, accurate inputs can get large reactions. This enables one to gather information about core material with an ease and speed impossible any other way. Mindfulness is established by: asking for it, describing it if necessary, but mostly by: speaking and acting in ways which invite it, that is, slowly, simply, and directly, with focused concentration, and without tension or judgment.

In Mindfulness, Evoke Experiences

Evoked experiences in mindfulness are different from ordinary experiences in several ways. They are unforced, automatic, and spontaneous, and therefore, reflective of habits and core organizers. Evoked experiences are also unpredictable and so, informative, naturally interesting, and likely to have meaning. Connections can be noticed between the evoking stimulus and the experienced reactions. A second advantage for therapy is that with evoked responses in mindfulness, the responsibility for the experience is clear. The therapist is not blamed for evoking a particular experience. The client does not feel "done to." Mindfulness allows the client to realize that he or she, on some deep level, creates the particular reactions. Of course the way the therapist goes about evoking experiences must be unquestionably nonviolent.

The ways we evoke experiences in mindfulness are given in the chapters which follow. I'll just name them here. They are: probes of all kinds, verbal, tactile, and visual, acknowledgments, taking over, and little experiments. The techniques are of little use without the training and skills to use them. Evocation depends more upon the state of mind of the client and the relationship between client and therapist than it does upon technique. We work with eight different kinds of experiences that are evoked: images, thoughts, feelings (from mild to overwhelming), sensations, memories, impulses, tensions, the child. When feelings overwhelm the client, we treat that as a processing state. When the child is evoked (covered in chapter 11), that too is a state of consciousness and, in that state "the child" is also having an experience of some kind, a feeling, sensation, etc. We may begin to work directly with the child.

Table 1. Transitions to Processing

EXPERIENCE EVOKED	EXAMPLES OF POSSIBLE APPROACHES
images	deepen with questions about details
thoughts	take over, find bodily experience
sensations	ask deepening questions
memories	get details to intensify and stabilize
impulses	active taking over
tensions	repeat, make voluntary, go for meaning
the child	use "working with the child" methods
mild feelings	use to access memories or strong emotions
strong emotions	use "riding the rapids" methods

The Transition to Processing

Evoked experiences are the raw material of processing. A transition to processing is the next step, once significant experiences have been evoked. The basic method for making this transition is: to find a way to stay with a the experience long enough for it to develop into one of the processing states. Staying longer than usual with an experience can mean anything from a few seconds longer to a minute or more. Some ways to stay longer are: simply wait, without interfering, and see if the client stays spontaneously; or, if there is some confusion or uncertainty, do some clarifying (perhaps by repeating the evoking process); or ask some deepening questions, that is questions directly about the experience itself. We can also make the transition by using accessing methods to establish one of the processing states directly, for example, by talking to the child or going for meaning. Each of these methods is covered in the chapters that follow. Techniques like taking over, probes, and doing little experiments are all used to make transitions.

The child state or strong emotions can arise at any time. When they do, they take precedence. So, even though going for meaning appears as a final approach in most cases, emotions and the child occur more often. In addition, all these states can change during processing. For example, in the course of going for meaning, strong emotions may emerge, followed by processing in the rapids for awhile and a final return to meaning.

State-Specific Processing

State-specific processing is similar to state-specific memory. We work with three different states of consciousness: strong emotions, the child state, and going for meaning. Going for meaning is not an activity of the intellect. It is allowing unconscious connections to be brought into consciousness. This is very similar to using mindfulness. It is passive and receptive, rather than active or analytic. We might, for example, ask this kind of question: "what does your body seem to be saying when it tenses like that?" We might also instruct the client not to try to figure it out but to let something come up by itself. There are different methods for each specific processing state, but the goals are the same. The methods are: for strong emotions (or riding the rapids): support spontaneous behavior. Here, we mean the spontaneous tensions and postures the client uses to manage his or her emotions. We usually support by using active taking over. For the child, we use a method called, "the therapist as magical stranger." That's covered in the chapter on working with the child. For going for meaning, we work at mind-body interface, going back and forth between the nonverbal experiences and a spontaneous, verbal expression of those experiences.

The goals of this processing are: emotional release, understanding and a change in the core organizers of experience. One way to reach these goals is to create an experience that wants to happen, an experience that couldn't happen because core organizers would not allow it. Such an experience often starts with riding the rapids or the child, progresses through meanings to the new experience, and ends up with deep feelings of satisfaction, relief and pleasure. It is accompanied by, or on occasion followed by insights and new understandings. The process continues then to stages of integration and completion.

The Best Leader

> *Learning is pursued through daily addition;*
> *Tao is practiced through daily subtraction.*
> *Keep on diminishing action.*
> *When nothing is pursued through action,*
> *Nothing remains undone.*
> *To win the world, one must renounce all.*
> *If one still has one's own ends to serve,*
> *One will never be able to win the world.*

- Lao Tzu, Tao Te Ching[2]

Many people do not mind if their therapist is directive. They want instructions and suggestions. Therapy is easier that way for them. The model we all carry for therapy or healing encourages a problem-solving posture, one in which the client presents a problem and the therapist, through questions, tests, advice and procedures, solves the problem. This model works well for many situations, like broken arms. But not (if you'll forgive a small, poetic liberty) for broken hearts. For working with deep feelings and painful memories, for working with the hurt, vulnerable and frightened child within, tests, questions, advice, and procedures are of little value.

For that, patience is needed, patience to wait for, and wisdom be led by, the other's unfolding. When the other is open and vulnerable, what happens next is not predetermined. What unfolds in those situations is strongly influenced by the conditions surrounding the very moment of unfolding. This kind of freedom isn't present all the time.[3] The freedom to change at the level of identity, to change who you are, happens rarely, during very special moments. These moments are made possible, in part, by something about the therapist. It is this: the therapist is extremely sensitive to what is happening within the other's experience, especially

THE FLOW OF THE PROCESS

BEFORE MOVING INTO PROCESSING

MANAGE THE PROCESS	STAGES	GATHER INFORMATION

by: by:

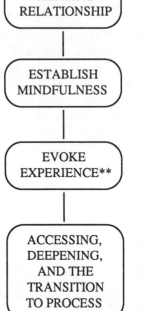

staying in the principles, getting the cooperation of the unconscious	CREATE A HEALING RELATIONSHIP	tracking*, empathy, following the story-teller, not the story
slowing down, turning inward, relaxing, focusing on present experience	ESTABLISH MINDFULNESS	tracking other's state of consciousness, stillness, inwardness
acknowledging, probes, taking over, little experiments	EVOKE EXPERIENCE**	track results of experiments, etc., track experiences evoked
accessing, deepening, probes, taking over, taking over voices, going where the other's unconscious takes you	ACCESSING, DEEPENING, AND THE TRANSITION TO PROCESS	track changes in other's states of interest, emotion, and consciousness

  * The things we track are: present experience, content, style, systematic behaviors, patterns of interaction, and signals from the unconscious.

** The experiences we evoke are: thoughts, feelings, images, memories, sensations, tensions, impulses, and the emergence of the child. These are the same as the present experiences we track for.

STATE SPECIFIC PROCESSING

GUIDELINES

get words for
experiences
and / or deep feelings,
clarify memories

be a compassionate
adult or take on the
role of Magical
Stranger

support spontaneous
behavior, especially
the management of
experience

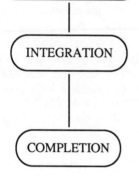

help create the
experience that wants
to happen

support the connections
being made, offer your
own, let client spend
time inside doing this

track for other's coming
to completion spontaneously,
use completion techniques,
if necessary

* Sometimes called Riding The Rapids

those signs that indicate where the process wants to go that it has never gone before. Not all processes are alive like that. Some are automatic, full of unconscious, habitual actions. In some, conscious choice is overwhelmed by feeling. In some, the flow of events is stopped by too much fear. Being controlled, overwhelmed, habitual or unconscious, these processes contain nothing new; no new feelings, experiences, insights or learning. They won't create deep changes. For that, something different must happen. The therapy must come to a moment of real choice, felt and deliberate. For the client to make real choices, the therapist must be following, not leading. The course of unfolding events must be conscious and directed by the deepest levels of the client's being. At these times, direction by the therapist interferes.

The essential process depends always on the therapist's ability to create a special atmosphere for the client. The client must feel that the therapist is following what he or she, the client, is doing, needing, or wanting. At whatever stage the process is, what happens next must be in line with what the client's deepest self agrees to.

Notes for Chapter 5

1. A Rolfer, Jeff Maitland, called it, "willful passivity." Relaxation, going along with the process, and staying with present experience are a very potent combination for healing.

2. Concord Grove Press edition, New York, 1983.

3. See Ilya Prigogine's "The reenchantment of nature," Chapter 10, in Dialogues with Scientists and Sages, Renee Weber, New York: Routledge & Kegan Paul, Inc., in association with Methuen, Inc., 1986.

6

CONTACT, TRACKING AND ESTABLISHING MINDFULNESS

INTRODUCTION

Contact and tracking are both skills and basic tasks. As skills they are needed throughout the entire process. As tasks they are especially important in the beginning, when we go about creating a healing relationship. As with everything else in Hakomi, they are also expressions of the principles. Tracking is the skill of following the flow of the other's present experiences. It is the constant seeing and listening in order to keep track of what is happening for the other. It requires an ability to get out beyond one's self and continuously stay with what someone else is feeling and doing. It is the constant reading of signs, as in tracking an animal through the woods. It is locking on and staying with the target, as in tracking a plane with radar. It is a way of being with someone, an attitude of interest and curiosity. It is not about the content of the other's story. It is not solving problems or figuring out who the other person is. It is much simpler than that. Therapy cannot proceed without it.

Contact has several levels: it is the task of creating a connection, as in "making contact"; and the task of maintaining that connection, as in "staying in contact"; and the skills with which all this is done; and, at the level of technique, it is a contact statement. The healing relationship is much more than just making and staying in contact. Still, the relationship requires that these tasks be handled. The tasks in turn require the skills to carry them out. One of these skills is the ability to create and use contact statements. Being in contact is something that we work to create. By analogy, we can think of receiving and sending messages back and forth. If we are in good contact, the messages flow smoothly. I know you are receiving me and you know I am receiving you. Communication trips gaily along.

As contact breaks down (like, static on the line), we have to repeat ourselves. Words are misheard. Understanding becomes difficult. When you see things like repeated and misunderstood statements in a therapy session, you can be sure that the process will not move on until contact improves. On the other hand, as one becomes skilled in tracking and making contact statements, communication improves dramatically. When these skills are fully matured, good communication is almost guaranteed.

The establishment of mindfulness is a basic task, essential to the flow of the process. It depends to a large extent on good tracking and contact. It also requires both the ability to communicate with someone in a non-ordinary state of consciousness and the ability to communicate the feel of that state to the other. This is done by being close to mindfulness yourself and conveying that through shifts in pace, tone of voice, speech patterns, and the kinds of words used. At times, images are also used.

Contact

Creating A Connection. Here's a simple example of creating a connection: I am working at a crisis center and a woman comes in. She's talking very rapidly. She looks and sounds very anxious. I'm sitting at my desk and she sits down in the chair next to it and she is talking non-stop about cars in the street and kids playing there and that it should be made into a play street and on and on. A big, long sentence. She never looks at me. She looks at the floor. She doesn't seem to want a response from me. She goes on talking, as if to herself. After a long while, she stops for breath. At that point I lean a little towards her and say clearly, "it's scary, isn't it." She looks up at me and into my eyes, until something inside her is satisfied, and then answers softly, "yes, I'm scared." Okay. Now, it's a two-person conversation. Now, she's talking to me and I'm talking to her. We've made contact.

To create a connection, the therapist demonstrates understanding. In the beginning, that often means following the details and import of the client's story. But, there's a catch there. If you demonstrate too often that you are following the story, the client will assume that it is the story you are interested in. You will get a lot of story that way, but the client isn't likely to go very deeply into his experience. For that, therapist and client have to focus on experience and experience only happens in the present. So, it is more effective if the therapist demonstrates understanding by showing that he is in touch with what the client is doing or feeling at that very moment. From both of these, following the story and following present experience, the therapist helps the client to feel heard and understood. Understanding has to be demonstrated. Just saying, "I understand," or going , "Uh huh," won't do it. The connection is also made by conveying to the client that this is his time. Mostly this is done by waiting. As the client talks, the therapist listens and watches, waiting patiently for the client to finish and signal that he is ready for the therapist to say something. Then, when the client is listening that way, the therapist can offer a contact statement. (See the section below.)

The therapist doesn't have to make a contact statement, certainly not every time the client stops talking. Contact statements are not mandatory. They are optional. Creating a connection is mandatory. And for that, one good contact statement may be enough. Nor does the therapist have to understand everything about the client to make a contact statement. It will be enough to understand some part of what the client is presently experiencing. The client is doing a lot of things all the time. Maybe the client is having trouble figuring something out. The therapist says something simple about that, like, "confusing, huh." It is not necessary or advisable to clear up the confusion. Just name it and see what the client does from there. Offering a short, simple comment on the client's present experience, shows that the therapist is following what's going on for the client. That's what does it! When that happens, the client often feels relief and safer. Feeling listened to and understood, the client relaxes and goes deeper. Good contact is rarely experienced outside of therapy. When it happens in therapy, it goes a long way towards creating the conditions for the cooperation of the unconscious and the unfolding of the client's process.

Staying in Contact. Most of what's going on in our experience is only passing through short-term memory. It can be lost in a moment as thoughts, feelings and sensations go rushing on. Present experience lasts only so long, if a mood or feeling changes, it may be available to consciousness only a few brief seconds more. Then, like last night's dreams, it's gone forever. If you're going to focus on something in particular, you must create a contact statement and use it while it is happening or within three or four seconds after it starts to fade. I was driving to Albuquerque with a friend of mine who had been studying Aikido for six or seven years. She was nice and relaxed when a loud noise suddenly happened behind and to the left of us. In response, she simply brought her left hand to about the level of her belly, held it flat, palm down, and unhurriedly turned her whole body toward the sound. The movement took less than five seconds. It was graceful and contained, a beautiful example of turning to face whatever it is that's coming, called in Aikido, irimi[1]. I watched, fascinated. I didn't speak for maybe thirty seconds. Then I asked her if she knew what she had done in response to the sound. She couldn't remember at all. She'd been focused on the conversation we'd been having and hadn't followed her own, beautiful movements. Years of training were in it and it had become habit. But, if in the first moment I had said, "Doing some Aikido, huh," the whole thing would have flooded into her consciousness, probably with a smile of self-recognition. Contact is made by going slow quickly. The feeling is relaxed and comfortable, but the timing is crucial.

Once created, the therapist maintains contact by staying attuned to the client's needs and pace and demonstrating that. For example, letting the client talk until you get a signal of some kind, usually a look, that it is okay for you to speak. Or being silent, while the client is inside, doing something like thinking, remembering, whatever. Or, the therapist uses contact statements to demonstrate that he is aware of moment to moment changes in the client. For example, when the client starts to feel something like sadness or pleasure. At those transition points, from one feeling to another or one activity to another, contact statements can be offered. Although the client may not comment upon these statements and may not even notice some, they have strong influences on the course of the process. To maintain contact, sensitivity to pace and transitions continues. The number of contact statements need not be many. The better the connection made and maintained, the fewer the contact statements needed to keep it going.

Contact and the Flow of the Process. It is especially important to leave time for the client right after offering a contact statement. In the moments after a contact statement, the client is becoming aware of something. Perhaps it is the sadness you've mentioned, or the conflict you've named. It is in these moments that the client, consciously or unconsciously, chooses which way to go. To stay with the new experience, to cry with the sadness, to call up memories, to move with his process or not. You must give the client room to do these things. It is the most important part of pacing and a strong signal that you are supporting what the client needs and wants to do. So, it's simple: after a contact statement, wait and see which way the client goes with it. For example: I listened to a client describe at length two parts of herself. Three to four minutes worth. I followed the details, but I didn't comment on them. I just said, when she had completed and looked at me, "So, two parts, huh." Simple-minded, you say. Yes. But it had this effect: she started crying. Not out of frustration because her therapist was an idiot, but because the split in her was deeply painful and that pain was what she was really presenting. I could have said, "painful, huh." Or, "a conflict, huh." She might have cried as easily at those. In effect, I summarized the situation she was presenting. I waited. She decided to let her feelings about the situation come through. It may not have been a conscious decision. It may have felt spontaneous. But, it must be a decision on some level. I did not make her cry. I only influenced that decision by demonstrating that I had understood her situation and by waiting to let her do what she wanted to do next. And she cried.

Influence is the right word. A contact statement allows the therapist to have a particular kind of influence on the flow of the process. The therapist is not directing the client to do anything, so, he doesn't evoke resistance. Yet contacting influences what happens. A contact statement about sadness says, in effect, "I notice you are sad and I'm interested in that." The silence afterwards says, "I'm listening, if you want to pursue that further." It comments and leaves space for the client to go where he wants to go with it. It helps create cooperation and make a two-way process out of the therapy. It allows the therapist to become part of the client's world, to enter into and participate, without creating a battle for control. Control ultimately belongs to the client.

Contact moves the process along by demonstrating that what is being expressed is understood. As in an ordinary conversation, a demonstration of understanding allows the speaker to proceed with the next thing he wishes to convey. Any lack of understanding and the speaker will try to make the same point again, possibly in another way. Or the speaker may simply give up, change the subject or walk off. In therapy, it is the whole process that needs to move along, from relationship, to mindfulness, to experience, to processing, to the experience that wants to happen. Experience needs to go from being talked about, to being felt, to being studied, to being expressed, to being understood. A contact statement like, "sad, huh," may be all that's needed to allow a moment of faint sadness to become a strong feeling and free expression. By showing that you know the sadness (or whatever) is there and by accepting it, you give it room to happen. For some people, especially people who feel misunderstood, good contact statements touch them and comfort them. That's a third purpose of contact. It lets the client know that he is not alone, that someone else is there who might just be able to help deal with the situation.

Contact also allows the therapist to focus on those parts of experience that are at the edge of consciousness. The hint of sadness that the therapist notices and mentions may have been just outside of consciousness. Mentioning it brings it into focus and allows something to happen about the sadness. Often this new focus is more exciting than the topic of conversation and replaces it easily. The process then has a chance to deepen. This is a small way of jumping out of the system, a part of the method we'll focus on later in chapter 18. It is also good practice for the client, who will have to learn about his own systems and how to jump out of them. It is the therapist though who jumps first, from the well-worn roads of ordinary conversation to the more fertile ground at the margin of the moment.

Meta-levels. There are two aspects to the overall interaction between client and therapist: content and form. Content usually remains figure, while form is part of the ground. From the content, you get the client's story. He tells you about himself. As part of listening to the story, you may get some ideas about what is going on at deeper levels, what kind of childhood the client had, what character patterns are being expressed. In the early stages of a session, you may listen to the story without interfering, establishing a few items of interest. While you may be interested in the quality of voice, the body structure, facial expressions, and posture, you are also learning about ideas, beliefs, assumptions and events in the client's life.

Though content is important, the form of interaction has much more influence on the course of therapy. The form of the exchange operates at a meta-level of communication, outside the content and usually outside awareness. It is established by the little things that go on. Things like who speaks first, who interrupts, who sits where, and all the many little gestures and extra-verbal happenings that control the flow of communication and make silent comment on who we think each of us is and what kind of relationship it is we're having. A few particulars:

By indicating that you're listening, you validate the other. You are saying with your attention that you recognize the reality of the other's experience, that you are willing to give them room to find all of themselves by offering the parts to you. You are not discounting or ignoring these parts as others may very well have done. By saying something back about the mood, feelings, and experiences of the other, you place these in the realm of material to discuss, while at the same time giving them a joint reality. A statement like "You seem a little nervous to me," offered without judgment and without breaking the rhythm of the other's presentation, is a way of making feelings real, okay to have and okay to talk about. Talking openly about whatever needs talking about and having your feelings, whatever they are, is often something that needs to be made okay. By going with whatever is going on for the person you're with, by letting them be, by supporting their taking the lead, if they will, you help them learn to run their own show. So, let whatever they're into be okay. If they are silent, meet them in their silence. "It's hard to talk about, isn't it?" That's the kind of response that will make it easier for them to begin talking again. Your own desire to "get things done" can wait. Meet them where they are. Think of it as, house calls.

Since the task of therapy, for the client, is to go deeply within and find the core of self, a big part of the therapist's job is to make it safe to do that. The highest responsibility the therapist has is to protect the spirit, the sense of hope and the life force. You do that by being safe yourself, by being nonjudgmental, accepting, and by keeping the situation safe. Contact is a very safe way to intervene and its use conveys that. Also, by talking about, looking at, and sometimes working with the body, we establish its place in the therapy. The whole idea of the body reflecting mental life is new to most people. So our ideas and way of working with the body have to be made clear. Of course, it is important to establish also that it's okay to have and express strong feelings—especially feelings that are considered "bad," such as anger, hate, envy, etc. These are faculties of the personality, talents, natural products of our natures. We are entitled to all of them, their opposites and then some. Support and accept all feeling and expression. Just make it safe and satisfying. Finally, in the early phases of the relationship, client and therapist establish how they will play their roles. Therapist's and client's ideas about that can be very different. Contact can help pick up these differences without creating conflict.

Contact and Aliveness. Effective therapists (and successful group leaders) know how to go where the excitement is. The level of excitement the client is showing is one of things experienced therapists habitually register. Highly charged issues get special attention. Contacting these moves the process towards work that is waiting to be done. The therapist can also wait for the excitement before showing interest, with a contact statement, perhaps. As Fritz Perls put it, "the emergency emerges." The way to use the available excitement is just to focus on it when it's there. Contacting charged issues before they are even mentioned is an easy way to engage the unconscious. A statement like, "take all the time you need," when offered to someone who has always felt pushed and hurried, will usually evoke an immediate interest.

Contact Statements. When the therapist offers a simple direct statement about the client's present experience, without interpreting, that's a contact statement. Something like, "sad, huh," when the client begins to show some sadness, is a good example. As we've already discussed, the statement can be about content or present experience. Some examples of contacting the content:

client talks about:	contact statement:
doubts, uncertainties	lots of questions, huh.
all he did for the family...	you really tried to help, huh.
something on his mind	so, that's interesting to you, isn't it.

Some examples of contacting present experience:

see:	contact statement:
tears, moist eyes	sad, huh. or, some sadness now, huh.
surprise	that surprises you, huh.
confusion	hard to understand, huh.

We've also noted that a contact statement can either refer to something the client is already aware of or it can refer to something just outside of awareness. Here's an example of referring to something on the periphery of awareness: Say the client is getting emotional talking about something that happened to him last week. Instead of saying something like, "Oh, that must have been hard for you," a statement which stays in the past, you contact the present experience. "A lot of feeling about that, huh." Meaning, "I notice you're having some strong feelings right now. Let's focus on them." Or, say the client is struggling to find words for something. "Hard to talk, huh." Those contact statements address something that's happening in the present but isn't being discussed.

Contact statements are usually short and simple. That way they avoid taking the client out of his process. They are also easier to create and more likely to communicate directly with the unconscious. Experiences are often one-word affairs, words like sadness, anger, confusion, and hurt. Short and simple though they may be, contact statements can be very subtle and intuitive; they can make big leaps from what's being said to what that all adds up to. A statement like, "feeling abandoned, huh," can seem to come from out of the blue and yet be exactly what the other is feeling. Or, contact statements can be low risk deals and totally obvious and still be very effective. When the client is inside working, not talking (and stops and leaves space for the therapist) the therapist can say some simple thing like, "something's going on, huh." And the client starts talking about it. Simple, but it works. It keeps the process going where it wants to go.

A contact statement must be given in such a way that leaves room for the client to disagree. Not that we want disagreement; too much of it disrupts communication and can ruin the cooperation of the unconscious. When you're making contact, you don't start an argument about who's right. Whose experience is it anyway? The client is automatically right. Even when you're sure you're right, and the tears are streaming down the client's face. If he says "no, I'm not sad," there's no argument. (Lao Tzu: better to retreat a mile, than win an inch.) Better to win cooperation and create safety than a stupid, minor point along the way. So, the therapist must be willing to be wrong and convey that through the delivery. You can't say, "I may be wrong, but..." every time. It has to be part of the way the statement is offered. And that has to happen consistently, with every statement. That means it must be part of the therapists unconscious attitude. If it is not, contact statements won't work well. It can't be a question, either. A question, even in the tone of voice, demonstrates that the therapist doesn't know something, isn't in contact. It may demonstrate interest and even caring, but it doesn't convey "following",[2] as in, "I'm following what you're saying." If I demonstrate that, you go on. If I demonstrate that I need more information, you start working for me in a way. Then the process bogs down. Whose process is it anyway. Too many questions and the client just waits for the next one and the next one, like an interview, and nothing spontaneous unfolds.[3] Contact is about moving the process along. Questions also invite thinking and distance, whereas contact statements invite experience and intimacy.

If we're making contact statements, we're not busy offering explanations or theories. We're not giving advice or asking questions (heaven forbid)! Those things create entirely the wrong impression. We're just trying to demonstrate that we're with the person, aware of their experience, following the flow of their process. Not just the client's words. The words are secondary. Experience is primary. I want to emphasize this strongly because, though it sounds easy, it's not all that easy to learn.

Tracking

...is looking for signs of the other's present experience, like moist eyes, all kinds of facial expressions, tone of voice, gestures (small or large, but especially small), changes in posture, movements, even the style of a movement or a voice. Signs of the other's experience. We learn to read them and we read them continuously throughout a therapy session. That's tracking. The signs can be very subtle. In ordinary conversations, most are missed or dealt with outside awareness. In therapy, they are a language that the client constantly speaks and the therapist constantly listens to. Without fluency in this language, consistently good contact statements are impossible. Tracking is noticing (following, again) all the little things that go on while someone is talking, especially the things that aren't being talked about. It is knowing how to read these as clues to the speaker's present experience and meanings. There's a great deal of very useful information in the things going on outside the words. Ask any serious poker player. These outward signs make comment on how the speaker feels about the things he's talking about. They express in body language, what is not being expressed in words. They are even more than just signs of present experience, they are direct expressions of the unconscious. The therapist has this two-fold task: to be in the world of the client, in all the usual ways, and at the same time, to be outside that world, able to see it from a wider perspective. Tracking is continuously following the whole person, conscious and unconscious, and never breaking contact.

Tracking the unconscious prepares the way for contacting and interacting with it to create the healing relationship. A simple example. The person comes in and sits down and you notice they look tense and nervous. You say, "I guess this is a little scary for you, huh." The person might actually have been thinking of what to say, not actually conscious of the nervousness at that moment. When you offer you statement about it, the person becomes aware of it at that moment and knows, again possibly without thinking it, that you are aware of what they are experiencing. That's usually a relief to them. Usually. Especially if your voice indicates that you are sympathetic. That helps create safety and begins meaningful communication with the whole person. On the other hand, if you continuously focus on the content of the conversation, not seeing what's going on around it, unable to contact experience and feeling, the process easily becomes boring. Boredom, being a sign of intelligence, is a signal to the therapist that he has lost track of what's really interesting for himself and the other.[4] It is a signal to start looking for a way to jump out of the system, lest we doze off thinking we're awake. Therapy is kept alive by tracking what's really going on. Once mastered, it is an endless source of curiosity and incredible fun. The ability to track, stretches one's awareness to the edges of consciousness, what is felt and real and happening, but not talked about. Yet.

There are gestures, movements, inflections, and changes in facial expression that we track which happen very quickly. Sometimes, in less than half a second. They are there all the time. And almost all the time, we are unaware of them. Given this natural tendency to become entranced by the words, the therapist must develop the skill of tracking. That usually takes a while. It is not so much that it is hard to do. It is more that it is hard to remember to do it. It is much like mindfulness in that it is open and sensitive and not so much task oriented. If we are accurately tracking the experience of the client, we can make good contact statements. And with each statement we make, each technique we use, each little experiment we try, we track the client's reactions to what we have done. So, it is a little cycle. Track, contact, track the effects of the contact. How did the client move along after we did this or that. Contact that. And on and on, like ball bearings, easing the process along, with a minimum of friction and wasted effort. Going somewhere by following. Therapists who use skills like tracking and contact are like explorers or experimenters, keeping track of local details while searching out larger truths. Like hardy travelers making for the pole, our eyes are close upon the dogs, as we push for the horizon.

Tracking States of Consciousness. Some outward signs of the four states of consciousness are:

ordinary consciousness :

> client looks at the therapist
> eyes are open
> tone and pace are conversational
> emotions low or controlled

mindfulness :

> eyes tend to close
> speech becomes softer and slows down by half or so
> when speaking or replying to questions, the person
> in mindfulness remains quiet and slow and keeps
> their eyes closed
> all the features of a light trance are there
> lack of movement
> deliberate, studious style
> breath is gentle

the child state:

> the voice is childlike
> sentence structure simple
> facial expressions, gestures and body look younger
> person shy in a childlike way
> a sense of wonder

riding the rapids:

> excitement
> high levels of emotion expressed
> wavelike movements of the body
> labored breathing.

Establishing Mindfulness

A State of Consciousness. Before attempting to evoke experiences in mindfulness, mindfulness itself must be established. Mindfulness, you may recall from chapter 2, is a non-ordinary state of consciousness. It is an open, vulnerable state and requires a relationship in which safety and rapport have already been established. Prior to using techniques like probes and taking over to evoke experiences, several things must be in place. One is the relationship. The methods for creating the relationship, tracking, contact, gaining the cooperation of the unconscious, will already be in use. All the signs of cooperation will be there. Second, before I start working for mindfulness, I have a good idea about what the other's interest is at this time. I have an idea about what I'm going to do once mindfulness is established. I have an idea about what will evoke an interesting, meaningful experience. There's no point in evoking a dull experience.

Thirdly, I wait for the other to finish telling me what he has to tell me[5]. Even if I have a good idea about what to do, I want to understand as completely as possible and I want to give him time to finish. When the client is finished telling me what he wants to tell me, he will stop talking and wait for me to make the next move. The client may slow down and relax then, also. I also work and wait for that slowing down and relaxation. When all that is in place, I may ask him if he wants to work on this thing that seems interesting.

If he does, I ask him to turn inward, maybe close his eyes, relax and just notice what happens when I... and then I do a probe or an acknowledgment. I don't ask for mindfulness directly. I am asking for a turning inward. I say things like:

> *just notice... you don't have to do anything... you can just be*
> *open and let my words come in and notice anything that goes*
> *on in your experience... it could be a thought, a feeling, a*
> *sensation, an image... it could be a memory... it could be an*
> *impulse or a change in muscle tension... and it's all right if*
> *nothing happens.*

I talk like that for thirty seconds of so. I don't talk in a normal, conversational tone or pace. I match my pace and tone, and the words I use to the state of consciousness I want to evoke. I also do it when I work with the child or when I work directly with the unconscious. To match for mindfulness, I slow the pace down by half or more. I use a soft tone of voice, like speaking to someone already in a trance. I use precise, simple words and short sentences. In matching the client's pace, I am constantly tracking to see how relaxed and turned inwards the client is. I don't keep talking this way unless I see that the client is receptive and still. When in mindfulness, the client's body will be very still and there most likely will be some movement of the eyeballs, up and down, under the closed lids. I track for these and for signs that the client is interested and really listening, like a slight tilt of the head.

Occasionally, a client will have trouble getting into mindfulness. It's rare, especially if the relationship is good, the story is done and a point of interest is established. But, it does happen sometimes. Usually, the person can't relax enough to get quiet inside. Another therapeutic approach is called for: massage, exercise, diet, vacation, or something medical perhaps. It only happens rarely; to me, less than a dozen times in as many years. But, it happens.

Once mindfulness is established this way, we use specific techniques to evoke experiences. Techniques are covered later in this book. For now, it is enough to know that in the use of technique, nonviolence is the first principle. Violence will destroy mindfulness in all but the most unusual people. We expect that even brief moments of mindfulness will yield significant experiences. These evoked experiences that can be used to access emotions, the child state or core beliefs, memories and images. Or, they can be deepened to stabilize and enhance them. This is the transition to processing and is covered next.

Notes for Chapter 6

1. In "The Bear", by Richard Heckler, from Lomi School Bulletin, Winter, 1981, he says, "In Aikido, we sometimes say that the solution may lie at the heart of the problem or the energy of the attack may be its own resolution. We say this because there is an aikido movement that epitomizes this quality of turning towards or facing. It is called "irimi" and translates to "entering." When an irimi technique is called for, we train ourselves to move directly into the heart of the attack or situation. This entering movement is non-aggressive in the sense that it is done in order to blend with the problem of the attack and not to oppose or strike back at it. We move towards this incoming energy, whether it be a physical attacker or a verbal tirade, in order to experience it at its most essential place and from there work with it ... creatively."

2. In the Tao Te Ching, Lao Tzu says, "the best leader follows."

3. You can see I've got a thing for questions.

4. Douglas Hofstaeder remarks, the difference between machines and humans is: machines don't get bored. Fritz Perls said, "boredom is repressed excitement."

5. Occasionally, a client will have trouble finishing his story. In that case, jumping out of the system is called for. That's covered in chapter 17.

7

EVOCATION ONE:
PROBES AND ACKNOWLEDGING

INTRODUCTION

W hen the client is in mindfulness and turned inward towards present experience, we're ready to evoke an experience of some sort; after the other has told us what he or she wishes to tell us. When the other is ready to go inward and we have the cooperation of the unconscious, then it's our turn to gently take charge and go to work. If we have listened and have some ideas about how we might proceed, then we use either a little experiment, a probe, an acknowledgment or we take something over. We may combine these techniques in elegant combinations. We do something very simple. In any case, it will most likely be one of the techniques discussed in this and the following chapter.

You can't tell what actually happens in therapy by reading theories. Techniques are often more expressive of the spirit of the work than all the discussions of how and why they work. Theory becomes important when it is time to teach the work. Techniques, however, remain palpable, clinical fact. In Gestalt, for example, the techniques involve the use of awareness, the hot seat, giving voice to various "parts" of the personality, and the exploration of dreams and fantasies. These techniques express what Gestalt Therapy is about. They express: a faith in imagination, playfulness and creativity. They express: a love of intimacy and presence, of being real, of owning and giving voice to all of oneself. These are things that words like "retroflect" and "confluence" don't tell us.

In Bioenergetics, stressful postures and strong expression are encouraged. The techniques reveal a determination to be energetic (in the old sense of lots of action), to work hard and not to run from one's pain. Pushing for emotions and expression is about being real. In psychoanalysis, it's the couch, free association and work with dreams. There's a great emphasis on the person as symbol user, with hidden, guarded worlds controlling daily actions and thought. Also here, an emphasis on the one-way street of the doctor/patient relationship.

Probes, acknowledging, contact statements, little experiments, and the various forms of taking over are the main interventions in Hakomi Therapy. We use them extensively during therapy sessions. Just as mindfulness and nonviolence are its central principles, these are the core techniques. Without them, Hakomi Therapy would be impossible.

I gave my first probe spontaneously. Everything my client was saying and the way she was acting told me she felt like a bad person. I asked her just to listen to me and to see what happened when I said the next thing. What I had in mind was her noticing her reactions to hearing me tell her she was a good person. I wanted to see what would happen. She had never said directly that she was a bad person; this seemed a habitual self-concept, not directly expressed.

I made a little production out of it. I asked her to look into my eyes, to let herself be open to my words and notice anything that happened. I watched her eyes to see when she was receptive. Then I said, "you're a good person." I said it slowly and more or less as if I were merely offering a fact. I wasn't trying to convince her, just offering the statement.

Now at the time, I was strongly influenced by Bioenergetics. I considered emotional release the primary goal of this therapy and I worked hard to bring it about, sometimes putting people through physically painful processes. I had the notion that emotional release was very hard to get. Well, when I said, "you're a good person" to her, she burst into tears and cried as I'd never seen her do before. After a while, we talked about her feeling like a bad person.

I still hadn't realized that I had a new technique. I didn't use my second probe for another six months. Probes didn't become a consistent developed part of my work for another two years. (If I look for a forerunner to probes, I find the closest thing would be Jung's use of the word association techniques developed by Wilhelm Wundt.) The next probe, I delivered to a woman who, in her first session, told me that she was the eldest of ten children, had children of her own and had no man around. We covered this in the first ten minutes. I thought about the things she might have wanted to hear from her parents, when she was a child taking care of her little brothers and sisters. I got her ready the same way I had gotten the first woman ready, asking for bare attention and looking into her eyes for the window. (We don't look into people's eyes any more. Most people like to keep their eyes closed during probes.) I said to her, "I'd like you to be my little girl." It's what I figured she never got to be, somebody's little girl. She cried, on and off, the whole rest of the session. This was a strong woman, and one who needed to be.

We talked when she wasn't crying and she sat in my lap and put her head on my shoulder. She felt what she'd missed and had never gotten, a need she had been running from, something she had once decided she would never get. My hope was that with her new consciousness of this and some experience of what it might feel like, she would try again to have at least something like that, sometimes.

I liked what had happened. She had felt pain but it was the kind of pain that happens when one comes back to one's self. I thought about it as helping the unconscious become conscious. The rest of the history is foggy. Probes slowly became part of the way I did things. Later, as I began to teach people, the theory and the technique just seemed to be meant for each other and to have always been so. They were, but it was a marriage made slowly. By the time I woke up to the connections, it had all been going on for a while. The other main techniques, taking over and acknowledging, evolved just as slowly. There's much more about them later in this chapter.

I've been personally inspired by a handful of great therapists. Right here I'd like to mention two, Albert Pesso and Moshe Feldenkrais. I took workshops with them, read their books and I feel their ideas and techniques were of the greatest importance in the development of my own. Both Feldenkrais and Pesso study the organization of experience, and both use mindfulness in their own ways. From Albert Pesso I learned to experiment and to allow the client to use his or her awareness to discover the meaning of experience. I learned techniques that leave awareness and self-discovery with the client, while also leaving plenty of room for the therapist's educated guesses to help the process along. From Pesso, I learned the importance of keeping the therapeutic environment safe and nourishing. I can almost hear him saying, "What happens when... " in his soft, attentive way. He was always creating, finding ways to structure the situation so that the client could make his or her own discoveries about what was right for them and what was nourishing for them. He was a master at this and I learned it from him.

PART 1:

PROBES

A probe is an experiment in mindfulness, an example of evoked experience, assisted meditation, if you like. We take time to prepare. We set up mindfulness, introduce a stimulus and study the reaction. We're looking for clues to the organization of experience. We ask the client to notice what happens, to note his or her reactions. When the client notices reactions and is able to report on them, the client is not reacting, but is in fact, responding, for noticing reactions is of a different order entirely from reactions themselves. With mindfulness, consciousness is self-reflective, able to study itself.

A probe is not conversation and it is not nourishment for nourishment's sake. We don't use probes when the client is in ordinary consciousness. It is an experiment, designed to evoke an experience worth studying and working with. With it, we hope to bring something automatic and unconscious into consciousness. We need mindfulness only for a brief moment. Probes are meant to evoke material to work with (See "Going Fishing," below) and to explore the memories and beliefs that organize experience.

Kinds of Probes

There are verbal and nonverbal probes: Verbal probes have this form:

1. Ask (if necessary, help) the client to become mindful.
2. Wait till the client is ready. (You can ask the client to signal you.) When the client is ready, offer a brief, simple statement. The statement part is almost always preceded by a question like:

> *Please notice what happens when I tell you...*
> *Please notice what you experience when you hear...*
> *What do you notice when you hear someone say...*

3. For people who are new at receiving probes and need some guidance, I extend the question part and use some of the same phrases for establishing mindfulness. In a slow, soft voice, I say:

Please notice what you experience... it could be a thought... a feeling... a sensation or an image... a memory might come up or some tensions in your body... It doesn't matter which happens; just so you're noticing. If nothing happens, that's perfectly okay... You can signal me when you're ready. I wait for the signal, and then...

So, please notice what you experience when I tell you...

This extended introduction helps get the client into mindfulness and conveys to the client that the mood is one of passive noticing and not effortful. After I deliver the probe, I track for the client's reactions to it. Statements like these are verbal probes:

What do you experience when I say...

you're a good person
I want you to be my little girl
your life belongs to you
you're perfectly welcome here
whatever you feel is okay
you are safe here
I am here for you

And on and on. The above probes, except for: I want you to be my little girl, are "generic." They have come up over and over again, in client after client. There are connections here between certain probes and the character processes that make just those probes hard to believe. Those connections are covered later in the book.

Nonverbal probes are similar, except that instead of offering a statement, the therapist performs an action, usually a gentle touch, or has the client do something, usually a slight displacement of the client's posture. When we select these physical interactions, touching and moving, we do it precisely and with mindfulness, they are very effective at evoking material to work with.

The Form of a Good Probe

Timing. We deliver probes slowly. Our pace serves as an example to the client; it sets the tone. We are doing things carefully, studiously. Our concentration acts to suggest the same to the client. Especially, it invites and supports mindfulness. You've asked for or established mindfulness and now, with your tone of voice and pacing, you're supporting it.

The Pause. There's a pause between the, "what happens when I say" part and the statement part of the probe. That little moment between the question and the statement allows the client to time the taking in of the probe precisely, especially after a bit of experience. If you're too abrupt, the client quickly returns to ordinary consciousness, reacting to the speed you're going and not the statement you make. So, go slowly and leave a pause between phrases.

Tone of Voice. As already mentioned, the tone of voice shows and suggests mindfulness. The tone is measured, careful, and neutral. The tone of voice avoids any effort to be convincing. It offers not the least bit of pressure to accept or reject the statement. Most people, especially when they are open and relaxed, will detect and react to even the slightest hint of coercion. So, the tone must be neutral.

Moreover, the voice must not go up at the end as it would with a question. A probe is a statement within a question and it is the statement that the tone of voice must emphasize. Questions automatically tend to shift consciousness to the verbal and away from experience. By avoiding the presentation of the statement part of the probe as a question, you help the client to simply notice reactions rather than think about answers.

Wording. The wording (given above), tone of voice and timing, help to structure the presentation of a probe as an experiment. With nonverbal probes, wording like this will work fine:

> *what goes on for you if I...*
> *what's it like for you when...*

A cautionary word about wording: avoid questions that ask for a particular mode of experience, like:

> *what do you feel when...*
> *what thoughts do you have when...*

Use broader terms than feel or think, unless you specifically want the thoughts, or a memory, or tensions. There may be times when you will want something specific. If the client dead-ends habitually in sensations or thoughts, you can ask for images or memories. But, if you're not looking for something like that, use words like experience, and happens, and goes on. The reason is simple. The client may not have a feeling when you do the probe. If you ask for feelings, the client will be looking for feelings and may not report other kinds of experiences. You give the client much more freedom when you use open words like, experience. Single Thoughts/Simple Language. You can't expect a short, simple, observable reaction to a probe when the statement in it is long-winded, complicated, intricate, or philosophical. The probe should be a single, simple thought. A five-year-old child should be able to be understand it. It must be delivered complete within a short time in spite of being spoken slowly, so you must not pause to think in the middle. Have it all ready to go before you even ask to do it.

Based in Reality. Don't try to sell the client a bill of goods. Don't go against the grain of what truly is, and was. Don't say things like: no one will ever be angry at you again. That's unrealistic and the client will have mixed feelings about it. Be realistic and truthful. If you're honest, as well as nourishing and accepting, you will have done your best and most likely you will also have done what the whole person, and especially the child within, needs and wants.

Nourishment. Probes should be nourishing or potentially nourishing to the client. We don't experiment with saying or doing things that are harmful or toxic. Sure, the client often feels pain when taking in a probe, but it's old pain and much of it is brought on by the recognition that what the probe offers was very much needed and wanted and just wasn't there for the child and probably isn't there now for the adult. That kind of pain is the beginning of healing. With a probe, we offer nourishment; we give the client an opportunity either to take in something that's needed or to see clearly that he or she rejects what's offered. From there, we can explore how and why that nourishment is rejected. We offer precisely the nourishment that we think the client needs and wants most and will have the most difficulty taking in. That's where the growth potential is.

Tailor Made. Though we use many probes to go fishing and at least two or three dozen are somewhat standardized, the best probes are developed and refined in an ongoing session with one particular client. One I remember went something like this: "you don't have to wash the dishes if you don't want to." As you work with a client, you refine your probes and change them until they are right on the money. Often a very small difference in a word or two will create a large difference in reaction. Even though the final probe may be similar to one of the generic ones, the small variation may be very important to the client.

Avoids First Person. If possible, it's best to avoid first person statements like: "I love you." It's better to say something like: "You're lovable." Since the probe is part of an attempt to observe reactions, avoid anything that tends to make that observation more difficult. With first person sentences, it's very easy to fall into an interaction based on transference. The client starts acting as if you were in an ordinary conversation. If that happens, it's wise to make it clear that the probe is an experiment and not necessarily a true expression of your thoughts and feelings. The experimental attitude is crucial. It is at the heart of mindfulness and the transcendence of dead habits and painful core beliefs. So, one gains some distance on oneself. At the same time, the work is intimate. It is about painful, deep, old things that remain mostly beyond ordinary awareness. This combination, of open, self-observation and great intimacy is rare in the everyday world and one of the things that makes therapy therapy. Remember, also, that you're not trying to be anybody other than yourself. You don't take on the role of good parent or anything like that. You are offering a statement as part of an experiment. Don't get into being other people. That confuses and complicates things.

Avoids Negative Words. In your effort to make probes simpler and easier to absorb, it's a good idea to avoid words like: not, don't, no, etc. Change statements like: "there's nothing to be afraid of" to things like: "you're completely safe here."

Of course, the client may ask for a statement with a negative word in it. Then you use it. As a general rule, whenever the client asks for something specific, try to give it in the exact form requested. Otherwise, avoid negatives.

Getting Reports. Lastly, and most important, the probe is of a form that asks for a report. You asked, "what happens when" and you want an answer to your question. The goal is to observe reactions and report on them. So, be waiting for a report! If you don't get one, ask for it! For example, the client may simply answer you as if you were in an ordinary conversation and had simply made the statement casually. Say, for example, you start with:

What happens when I say... you're a good person?

And the client answers:

Well, nobody ever said that to me before.
Or: You don't really mean that.

When that happens, you'll have to ask for a report:

I understand what you're saying, but I don't think you told me what happened. Did you notice anything, a thought, a feeling, something?

Get a report! Usually, you try it again after clearing up the procedure. If the client gets stuck in reacting and not giving reports, you'll have to house keep that and do something to change the situation. Maybe demonstrate with someone else. Maybe try some more safety and relaxation stuff.

These are some of the aspects of the form taken by probes. With very little practice they are quite easy to deliver properly. The next thing to talk about is where we get them.

Creating Probes, From...

The Standard Set. Hakomi therapists have created and discovered dozens of probes over the last ten years. Most reflect character processes at one level or another. Three or four core beliefs and several more peripheral ones are associated with each character process. With the sensitive process, for example, beliefs around being safe and welcome are important. So, one probe used often with sensitive processes is:

You're perfectly welcome here.

In the early part of a therapy session, a standard probe can be very effective for going fishing (below).

The Body. One of the ways to discover which probe might work is to look at the client's body, including posture, structure, gestures and movement style. From such observations, you can make some judgments about which character processes you'll be dealing with in therapy. It's a matter of knowing how to read bodies for character information and of having the probes that go along with each process.

Content. The content of the client's story is a rich source from which to create probes. The client's world is constrained by assumptions and the meanings of important past experiences. By listening closely for the client's experience and its meaning for him or her, you can determine the beliefs that limit nourishment and well being. If the client is talking about how hard he or she tried to please her parents and you hear sadness and disappointment in her voice, you can try a probe like:

You don't have to please anyone but yourself.
Or: You're lovable just the way you are.

Those are standard probes for the rigid process. A wonderful suggestion from Pat Ogden is: imagine what type of statement would make good contact and turn it into a probe. For example, you can transform a contact statement like: "tired, huh," into a probe like: "it's okay to rest."

Metacommunications, Like Tone of Voice

All kinds of things are going on that silently comment on the content of the conversation. Gestures, facial expressions, and the tone of voice all yield clues about what is going on for the client and are therefore, potential sources of probes. For example, a tone of voice that indicates a questioning, uncertain attitude. Every sentence ends with the voice going up, as if it were a question behind every statement made. That's a clue to character and often is about being understood. So, a probe that might work would be:

I hear you and I understand.

That probe is related to processes about getting attention and being loved, like the expressive/clinging process. By the way, you can also transform probes into acknowledgments, like this one about understanding could be transformed into:

I know you need me to listen and understand.

So, tracking the client's experience and mental processes is essential and primary. From tracking, you can make contact statements, acknowledgments or probes.

The words the client uses are also clues: A statement like, "I never get what I want" would most likely elicit from me, at the next opportunity: What happens when I say... you can get what you want?

It's not that I'm ornery. There's a lot to discover about how one organizes oneself around such a dismal belief. Memories directly related to such a belief may well emerge in response to using that probe.

From content, posture and tone of voice, a pattern emerges which makes sense of the client's whole experience. By listening, looking and experimenting with ideas in your mind, you discover what's going on for the person you're working with. After a little practice, or a lot, probes come effortlessly to mind.

The Connection to Principles, Method and Process

The connection between probes and the principle of mindfulness is obvious. We are using our best tool for self-discovery. We are studying, using a special state of consciousness. We are exploring and noticing. Probes are one of the uses we make of mindfulness in Hakomi Therapy, and a clear expression of our commitment to that course. We are also being nonviolent. We are letting the clients discover for themselves. There's no force, no interpretation, no explaining the client to himself.

The reactions to verbal probes are often physical sensations, tensions, or movements, whereas the reactions to nonverbal probes can be thoughts, images, memories, etc. There is the flavor of holism about that, a constant crossing of the mind-body interface. In a paradoxical way, attention to one's reactions - which are, after all, very mechanical - contributes also to a sense of being alive and "organic." The part that notices, the part that is beginning to feel free to choose, has the sense of growing aliveness.

We use probes in different places within the process. They're very effective in the beginning, after the therapist has heard and seen the client for a few minutes and has an idea about what is going on. At that point, we use probes to evoke experiences to work with. I like to call that use of probes: going fishing. If you hear something in what the client is saying or see something about the way he or she sits, moves, etc, you can try a probe related to the material you suspect is there. Once you've gotten a strong, clear reaction, you can make any of several transitions to processing. Anything that happens in reaction to a probe can be useful in making the transition to processing. It also helps if you have inspired guesses about what the reactions mean. Then your next probe can be even more accurate and evocative. You have to know how to listen in order to create probes.

We don't use probes during strong emotional release or while working in the child state of consciousness. Those two processing states require direct physical and verbal interactions. They are not appropriate for work in mindfulness. While making the transition to processing, that is, while deepening or accessing, probes are very effective. They are also used to clarify behavior at the barriers of the sensitivity cycle. Varying the probes, exploring different aspects of the objections to nourishment and the reluctance to respond are all part of that clarifying.

PART 2:

ACKNOWLEDGING

A Transcript of An Acknowledgment

Therapist: I don't know what you want to do about this sadness.
Do you want to find out what kind it is or do you want to find out what it's doing here now?
Client: (Still showing a very sad face, nods yes on second possibility.)
T: Okay, so you want to find out what it's doing here now.
C: (Nods again.)
T: Okay. So, I want to ask the sadness a question. You don't have to answer it yourself. You can just wait and see what the sadness will answer. Okay?
C: (Nods yes.)
T: Okay. So, I want to ask the sadness, "Sadness, what are you doing here now?
C: (Some small deepening of the sadness and...) It says, "I just want to be here."
T: Okay. So, it just wants to be here. Okay, I want to acknowledge that. I just want to say something to the part that's sad and I want you to just notice what happens when I say it. Okay?
C: (Nod. Still a lot of sadness showing.)
T: You signal me when you're ready!
C: (Slight pause. Nods readiness.)
T: Sad part, now I know, you just want to be here. (This is the acknowledgment, spoken in a gentle, slow voice, with the client in mindfulness.)
C: (Relief. Some deepening of the expression of sadness. Shifts to a more child state of consciousness.)

After this brief exchange, there's a clear feeling of a deepening connection between client and therapist. The child part, feeling alone and having difficulty expressing herself, finds someone there listening and becomes able to speak. An unfolding of the whole process begins. The client opens to the experience of needing to be there with her sadness and needing that to be okay with others. She starts to get in touch with never feeling she had that and believing that she would never get it. This acknowledgment has strongly shifted the relationship of client and therapist and of the conscious adult part of the client to her child part.

Some aspects of the client are in the shadow, ignored or denied, hardly ever shared with others. In the person's past, these general experiences were not acceptable to others and couldn't be shared. They were "put aside." The client may not acknowledge these experiences, even to him or herself. The experience is waiting to happen and it's full of painful memories, feelings and ideas.

In the transcript above, the feelings were about a sadness that was just there and seemed to have no explanation. Early in the session, the client just wanted the sadness to go away. It wouldn't. Her beliefs — we discovered shortly after the excerpt above — were that if she showed her sadness and let it be there, people would leave and she would be alone. The child part had decided that she would always be strong and not show weakness or need.

In this technique, with the client in mindfulness or sometimes, just with the unconscious present and listening, the therapist acknowledges a core experience which has been denied and is being re-experienced at the moment. The point is to say something to the unconscious that shows that you are understanding what it is trying to tell you. Such interventions are powerful. They establish the truth and admissibility of experiences that are: (1) real parts of the client; (2) close to the core; (3) have pressed for awareness and expression, without much success; and (4) have had no ally in the client's history. Something that was not, or could not be, discussed or understood, is now open again for consideration and someone has witnessed it, making it real and present.

Acknowledging builds the healing relationship by demonstrating real understanding from the therapist. It is done much like a probe, only it expresses a recognition by the therapist of some deep, long-term experience of the client. It is, "contact in mindfulness." I use it when I realize that the client has lived a long time with this exact experience. When acknowledged, this powerful, generic experience, part of the client's basic experience for a lifetime, emerges, deepens, and fully enters the present process.

So much now for probes and acknowledging. We move on to the other main techniques: taking over and doing little experiments.

8

EVOCATION TWO: TAKING OVER AND LITTLE EXPERIMENTS

PART 1:

TAKING OVER

From Moshe Feldenkrais, I learned about sensitivity and noise and about taking the effort out. The whole sensitivity cycle (Chapter 15) is an elaborate development of the Weber-Fechner Law, which he talked about in his first book, *The Body and Mature Behavior*. Though I'd known the law from my studies in psychophysics, I hadn't seen it's application in therapy at all. One of Feldenkrais' gifts was his ability to see the application of such things in the basic techniques of therapy. Not all minds can make such leaps. The whole idea of taking over derives from Moshe and the Taoist notion of supporting the natural flow of events. I learned this same special use of sensitivity and awareness directly from Moshe.

Taking over refers to a whole genre of techniques. In all these techniques, the therapist takes over doing something that the client usually does for herself. It's an offer to make things easier, to take some of the effort out of what the client is doing. If you're scratching your head, I can offer to do it for you. All you have to do is let me. You drop your efforts, like raising and moving your arm. Or, you could be saying things to yourself. I could say them for you. On all levels, taking over is an offer of support. It is an offer to participate.

The technique of taking over is a simple one. It involves, say, letting the client's head rest gently in your hand, taking the weight of it, when it falls forward with sadness. Or, if the client's reaction to a probe is an internal voice, we can take that voice over and say it for the client. There's a great variety of things we can take over, limited only by our own creativity. A small list is given below in the section called, Things We Take Over. For now, let's look at the effects. Taking over:

1. tends to support the need for safety
2. lowers the noise, thereby increasing sensitivity
3. helps create distance and control over reactions
4. supports the healing relationship
5. shifts awareness from defensive concerns to consciousness of the feelings, impulses, images and memories being defended against

By taking something over — the weight of the head, for instance — we provide an opportunity for the muscles which are holding the head in the forward position to relax. We don't make things happen; we provide opportunities. Letting the head fall forward is usually an unconscious action when it is part of the feeling of sadness. Its function is to help manage the experience of sadness and its expression. The weight of the head, acting on the muscles of the chest and back, makes it difficult to breathe deeply. (That's very easy to experience for yourself if you'll just try breathing deeply, first with your head back and then with it hanging over in front.) The effect of this limit on breathing is a limit to feeling.

But taking the weight of the head, the therapist takes over the work of those muscles; even with the head still in the forward position, the client can now breathe more deeply and will either do so, thereby deepening the experience, or will try to manage the feelings by taking back the weight of the head, or by tightening other muscles (the diaphragm, most likely).

When the offer to take over is accepted (by relaxing the muscles holding the head up) it has the effect of taking the effort out of an important reaction. Taking the effort out, lowers the noise. The noise of efforting masks experience. Tensions narrow experience. That's one of the ways people use tension and effort. Think of banging your finger with a hammer. The breath stops, the whole body tightens — to manage the experience of pain. When we offer to take over the client's efforts to manage his or her experience, we give the client an opportunity to stop managing, to relax the tensions involved, to become more sensitive and to deepen the feelings and experience being managed. Often, taking over actually brings blocked feelings into consciousness. It is a direct route to suppressed, repressed and otherwise managed experiences.

The first time I took something over was at a workshop in New Mexico. I was working with a woman who was getting very close to something important and charged with feeling. She was lying on her back on the carpet and, as we focused in on her experience, her back began little by little to arch. After a few minutes, her body was a bridge with only her head and her heels on the floor. I was still into bioenergetics then. My approach to defenses was to force them to yield. Since I saw the arching as a defense, I was prepared to put a lot of weight on the woman's abdomen until the bridge came tumbling down. In my mind, that would have been the logical, defeat-the-defenses approach. What could be more archetypically rigid than arching backwards like a bridge? I knew it was so because I'd experienced that same arch myself once. I remembered how involuntary it felt. It was just happening. I knew how terrible it would feel if I tried to make the client collapse. I couldn't bring myself to do it, even in the name of therapy. Instead, I put my hands under her back — and I told her that if she wanted to, she could relax her back and I would hold her up. It was my first time taking over, though I had no name for it then and wouldn't for a long time after. Well, she tested my hands a little, giving them some of the weight at first and then, little by little, all of it. This took a minute or less. As she let herself give the weight of her body to me, she also let herself feel and experience the things that she had been fighting against — a painful memory and the feelings and insights that went with it. She eased into that and we worked with it.　　Imagine if I had pushed against that arching. Imagine the struggle, with her caught between my pushing down and the unconscious forces within her pushing back. Imagine the chaos and effort and pain. What would be the result when she finally collapsed? We would have forced the insights into consciousness along with painful, chaotic feelings. She would also believe, correctly, that all this had been done to her (or as it is often put, for her). She would have expended her energies in fighting the therapist and bearing the pain. Any healing or integration would first have had to overcome the treatment.

But she didn't have to make that struggle. Instead, she let herself relax, slowly, at her own pace, into the experience she'd been running from. She saw it clearly. She processed it with awareness and, though she recognized the support I gave her, she quite rightfully took complete credit for facing and dealing with that painful experience in a new way. It was her accomplishment. She did it. I created the opportunity and she took it. That's what happened and that's what she experienced. For her, it was an empowering experience.

For me, it was a liberation. I began to see more and more ways to help clients without struggling against them - by helping them to do what they were already doing. I saw a way to step into the client's defensive maneuvers and, like an old Aikido wizard, help the energy go where it needed and wanted to go, without effort and without the ego-heavy role of doing battle with the unconscious.

A person arching or folding inward or clutching himself is trying to organize his experience in order to make it safer and less painful to deal with. When a therapist offers to help him do that, there is almost always a feeling of greater safety. The client feels supported, trusting. It's a matter of having someone on your side, someone who is giving you time to prepare and time to absorb. There isn't the underlying feeling that the therapist is judging you, looking, as it were, right at your disease and wanting to take an ax to it. Not having to deal with that lowers the noise and gives the client the strength and courage to face what needs to be faced. The therapist is not the frightening figure who will cause you pain "for your own good." The therapist is the support giver, making the work of self-discovery easier, safer and clearer. Therapy goes very differently when the client feels this way. This is the type of healing relationship that the unconscious can appreciate and participate in.

This combination of sensitivity and safety allows the client to shift identification from the part that manages, to the impulses and feelings being managed. When the therapist takes over these management reactions for the client, the client becomes free to be the other parts, the parts kept contained or out of awareness. This allows a shift in perspective and is a powerful way to access core material. The big, tough/generous person comes very quickly into contact with the sad, frightened child inside that he's protecting. The burdened/enduring person almost immediately feels the impulse to freedom.

Just imagine how freely you could express anger if people were securely holding you back. Or how satisfying it would be to try moving past a long, slow line at the airport, jump over the counter and to do mayhem and murder there, if six strong friends would be there to stop you. Think of all the lovely things you could say to the cop that just pulled you over if someone would just hold a hand over your mouth. Think of all the ways you hold yourself back and keep a hand over your own mouth and a veil over your mind.

You would shift in a moment, from mild-mannered Clark Kent to Superman. You could identify with your own aggressive impulses, where a moment before you were all caught up in holding them back and staying in control. It is now safe to express yourself. Someone else is holding you back. Someone has taken over your controls for you, your controls against expressing parts of yourself you have pushed into the shadow. You have become free to own them again and know them for what they are. In this safe situation, you get to feel and be parts of yourself you thought you lost and forgot a long time ago.

So, taking over promotes the movement into consciousness of material that has long been unconscious—a big step in changing habits to voluntary processes. I learned a lot about taking over from watching and reading Moshe Feldenkrais. It is his notion that almost all our movement habits are associated with being in the field of gravity. We organize the rest of our efforts around that central core. In order to re-organize, it is best to remove as much as possible this central organizing core. Thus Feldenkrais has people lie down, giving as much weight to the floor or table as they can. Or he puts towels and pillows under those spots where the body is too tense to relax into flat contact.

By this means he is simply taking the effort out. He is taking over the effort to hold the body up, or he's having the floor do that, so that a new set of habits can emerge. The organizing core, the response to gravity, is no longer needed and habits attached to that core no longer need be organized by it. They are free to be reorganized and reintegrated. In the same way, the automatic ways we manage core material, the holding in or holding back, the tendency to withdraw or persist, lose much of their power when we take the effort out of them.

In Chicago some time ago, I worked with a woman who was suicidal and self-mutilating. As soon as we met, I sensed how fragile she was. She wasn't small or anything. She had a large body, especially around the hips and pelvis, with a disproportionately small chest and thorax. As we spoke, I became more and more gentle. She was at the same time fragile and very tense, like a frightened bird, poised for sudden withdrawal. As we talked, she made a gesture, a movement of her fist towards her side. I asked her about it. She said she felt like stabbing herself. I decided to take over her holding herself back, so she could get deeper into trying to stab herself. She was obviously struggling inside with that impulse. So, I said, "okay, I'll hold you back and you try to stab yourself." I looked around for something she could use to stab herself with and found a nice big spoon. Something more like a knife would have been even better.

The moment I got a grip on her wrist, this quiet, tense woman started thrashing about in an effort to drive that spoon into herself. We fought till we fell to the ground, but we kept struggling and rolling around. I was pooped. I couldn't have held her back much longer. She didn't seem the least bit tired. She showed no signs of wanting to stop. She was, in fact, having the time of her life. Just imagine, after years of struggling with that impulse of wanting and not wanting to kill herself, after all the despair and fear and pain, of doubts, and thoughts of going to hell. After years of terrible constriction and control— she was getting a chance to let it all hang out. And that's just what she was doing. Maybe she felt safe enough, that I was a therapist and by definition knew what I was doing. That I was responsible.

It came to the point where I would have to stop. I was becoming exhausted. Given that demonic gleam in her eye, I didn't expect any sympathy. So, I mustered my calmest and most completely rational voice (the kind that is so completely reasonable, it simply does not enter one's mind to doubt it). I said to her, "let's stop for a moment." (I was also trying to act as if I had all my wind and strength left.) She looked at me with total disbelief. What did I mean, stop! Was I nuts? Did I think she could just quit this passion, abort this totally absorbing, completely carried away, murderous, delicious suicidal fit. Just like that? Was that what I thought?

I looked back into her disbelieving eyes without wavering in the slightest from my sweet, deceiving calm (which I was working hard to maintain). I was all steady reasonableness which made a silent but definite reply, "Yes, indeed, that's exactly what I think." Well, after a while the deadlock began to dissolve. She slowly relaxed and gave up the struggle. She transformed herself into a quiet, rational human being before my very eyes. We talked a while about her experience. Then, when I was rested, and because she loved it so, we took it up again. Same thing happened. Then we talked and rested. Then we did it again. The fourth time we stopped, she did it easily, without a lick of trouble, as soon as I asked her to.

She got well under the therapeutic care of her regular therapist and the next time I came to Chicago, six months later, I didn't recognize her. She had changed into a light, happy person. She had to explain to me that she was the woman who had been suicidal. My guess about what she got from our session was, for one thing, a much deeper understanding of her self-hatred and the direct knowledge that she could stop any time she wanted to.

The Forms of Taking Over

There are three basic dimensions to taking over:

> 1. with mindfulness and without
> 2. active and passive
> 3. physical and verbal

With Mindfulness and Without. With mindfulness, you use taking over just like a probe, to go fishing, to evoke material to work with. Without mindfulness, it is used during the spontaneous or overwhelming expression of strong emotions (riding the rapids). It is the basic way we support spontaneous behavior in that state of consciousness. During the rapids, we do not ask for mindfulness; we simply support anything the client does spontaneously to manage the flow of feeling. If, for example, the client curls up in a little ball, we help her to curl. If she wants to roll over, we help her. If she covers her heart, we put a hand there, too. Whatever she does to manage the flow of experience, we offer to help.

Active or Passive. Taking over is either active or passive. In the active version, we are asking the client to do something, to be active. We might for example ask a client to punch while the therapist holds the client's arm back. The taking over I did with the suicidal woman was active taking over. It involved an active struggle. In passive taking over, we ask the client simply to be passive. For instance, we might ask the client to relax and notice what happens as we slowly lift the client's arm or arms into a reaching-out posture. Or, if the client is doing something like covering his eyes, we might do that for him.

Passive taking over with mindfulness requires a high degree of sensitivity on the client's part. If the client isn't able to focus quietly and sensitively on what's happening, if there's just too much tension in the person, if there's too much need to move or work, then it's a good idea to use active taking over. Then, instead of searching for subtle meanings, you ask the client simply to find a way to struggle actively that feels good or right. Getting pleasure from using the tension in the body is a potent route to relaxing and becoming more sensitive.

Physical or Verbal. Lastly, taking over can be either verbal or physical. The above examples are all physical. A verbal taking over is one in which the therapist takes over a voice heard inside or a thought the client has in reaction to a probe or to the meaning of some physical tension. Some examples:

In Germany, my first trip over, a woman in my evening group was very agitated and looked very tired. I asked her about it and she told me she hadn't slept for several days. She had cancer of the stomach. I worked with her a little bit using probes and we discovered a terrible conflict about going to sleep. One side was a belief that if she slept, the cancer would grow while she was sleeping and would eventually kill her that way. Another belief, almost as strong, was that she must rest or she would grow weak and not be able to get well. I used was passive taking over. I asked her to lie down and relax as much as possible and just to notice what happened when.... And I got two people, one on each side of her, to repeat as precisely as possible, in the exact words and voice, the two sets of thoughts she'd been having. The two people worked a few minutes getting the sentences exactly right and then repeated them, over and over, both talking at the same time. After a hearing the first two or three sentences, she relaxed deeply, and in a few minutes she was fast asleep. In that instance, we took over a whole conflict. It was passive, verbal taking over.

Here's another example: Suppose you try a probe and the person's throat tightens. Then you ask the person to tighten it again a few times voluntarily, to get what the body is saying by tightening the throat. The client comes up with the words, "I won't cry!" Well, you ask the client to relax and just notice what happens when you quietly say it for them. You say, "I won't cry" a few times and the client may say something like, "My throat relaxed and I can feel my jaw trembling and there are tears in my eyes."

Any given instance of taking over has aspects of all three dimensions - verbal or physical, active or passive, with or without mindfulness.

Things We Take Over

Thoughts and Beliefs. As with the woman in Germany.

Muscle Tension. There are many ways to take over muscle tension. We use active taking over with chronically tight muscles that have a lot to do with posture. For example, when a person holds his or her shoulders high and tight, we take them in a circle grip, using our arms to hold them up and in, and we ask the client to try to force the shoulders down against our resistance. The struggle usually feels very good to the client. That's one of the signs that we're on the right track, that it feels good. After all, we are doing something for the client that the client has been doing for herself maybe all her life. In addition, by dropping the shoulders, the client may be expressing something that she has been holding back just as long.

Often, during an emotionally intense session, the client will suddenly feel a muscle tightening as his experience comes close to something significant. We can ask the client to relax the muscles involved while we tighten for them. For example, the abdominal muscles often become tight quite spontaneously during intense feeling. The therapist can use a hand or a fist to create pressure there while the client allows the muscles to relax. That's a passive taking over of muscle tension. I once took over, very slowly and precisely, the muscle tension of a headache. When I had simulated the tensions well enough, I ask the man to just relax and let me be the headache tensions for him. Slowly, he did. After a few minutes of holding, I asked him to direct me in taking my fingers off, one at a time, while he concentrated on not tensing up as we did that. In a few more minutes, I had taken my fingers away and his headache was "95 percent gone." Since he was a leading teacher of biofeedback, I figured he was probably no more than a few percent off.

Blocks to Expression. The safety of being contained allows an impulse that wants expression to emerge, perhaps for the first time in years, and with it comes realizations about how we've limited and controlled ourselves. This is especially true in relation to blocks to the expression of anger, rage and hate, and impulses to harm others. By holding back arms or by holding the jaw closed, the impulse to strike, bite, choke, etc, can emerge. Muscle tensions are often associated with such blocks to expression. The taking over is always voluntary, always guided by what the client wants and feels comfortable with. It always stops when the client wants to stop. It is never used as part of any provocation. It is done in the spirit of service. We do only what the client wants done. Control is always with the client. Without these safety aspects, the process never becomes spontaneous or goes very deep. It may be acted out, full of sound and fury — you know the rest.

Gestures. Many gestures involve self-touching. Without noticing it, people will often touch their chests, or cover their eyes, or clasp their hands together, or rub an arm or a leg or a neck. Any of these actions can be taken over. At first, the client may notice only that it feels good or that it makes her sad in a good way that you are touching her. But with a little time and mindfulness, the meaning of the touch can become clear. It represents, of course, something the client believes she has to do for herself but would be much nicer coming from someone else, like comfort and caring. I remember my father making circles with a hand on his chest. Standing there in the morning, eyes in the middle distance, rubbing his chest that way through his undershirt. I found myself, in my thirties, doing the same thing. I learned, in therapy, at age fifty-four, when a fellow teacher did that for me that it was all about reassurance. I needed my father, when I was small, to tell me everything would be okay. Just that. He couldn't do it. He needed someone himself. When Bill took over that movement, I felt first the sadness, then I cried, then I realized what it was all about. That's a typical sequence of events when taking over is used: an immediate experience, like a feeling or an image, followed by feelings and expression, followed or accompanied by insight.

Impulses. In cases where the client is very strongly identified with the resisting doing something (like striking out, for example), we can take over the impulse itself: "You make a fist and I'll try to get you to swing it and you resist. Let's see what happens when we do that." Often, the strong injunctions against showing anger come up along with memories of related situations. After a while, the taking over can be reversed, with the client trying to strike out and the therapist holding that back. Or you can go back and forth. When taking over in one direction is not productive at first, especially when the client's chronic tension level is high, we can alternate (like the shuttling done in Gestalt Therapy) between taking over the block and taking over the impulse.

Self-support. We've already mentioned Feldenkrais' decision to put pillows in the gaps between the body and the table. In any area where the client is holding herself up in some way, like propping the head on an arm or leaning back on a wall, etc, we can take over supporting the person. This way of taking over works very well with people avoiding letting down and needing to rest, because they feel no one is really there for them, as in the self-reliant or dependent endearing strategies. It is a good way to explore the blocks to taking in nourishment. The examples above give only things we take over and many more will be devised.

Taking Over, the Principles, and the Method

Taking over is a prime example of the Taoist principle of going with the grain and in a beautiful way, reflects the principle of nonviolence. It is nonviolence itself. By helping the client to do what he or she is already doing, we simply step into the flow of the client's experience safely in a way that supports. It speaks of respect and it honors self-determination. For me, it is the queen of techniques. For example. A woman called me once, from the infant massage, day care facility in Boulder. She told me they had a three-month old infant who, when touched would just bring his legs up over his head and would keep them there. He seemed not to want to be touched. I told her that when the infant did that, just help it by taking over the holding of the legs in that position. She called my back thirty minutes later. She'd tried it. After about two minutes of holding the legs there, the infant relaxed totally, his legs flopped open and he received what looked and felt to her like an thoroughly enjoyable massage.

I got another call once — from a woman whose twelve years old daughter had been raped in there own home during the night. The woman had participated in an introductory workshop with me some time before. She said she just wanted to thank me for teaching taking over to her. After the rape, her daughter couldn't sleep at night. She would stare at the door to her room and wouldn't turn the lights off. The mother talked with her — she was all sweet reasonableness and comforting — but it didn't help. Finally, she told her daughter, "I'll watch the door for you." She said she would sit there all night and watch the door for her and she wouldn't go away without telling her. After much reassurance, the daughter closed her eyes and fell asleep. "I'll watch the door for you." That's what did it. That's taking over.

In keeping with the overall method, taking over is primarily a technique for lowering the noise, thereby increasing sensitivity and gathering information not previously available. As mentioned above, we use taking over to explore experience and to evoke core material. We use it in all stages of the process. In relation to the sensitivity cycle and the barriers, we use it very deliberately. The different forms of taking over are useful in different degrees at the different barriers. Whereas active taking over is very appropriate at the response barrier, in helping to release impulses that want to happen but are held back, passive taking over works a lot better at the completion barrier, where the client needs to melt and to learn to let go. Taking over self-support is a good way to work at the nourishment barrier; helping to control information input, by taking over blocks to feeling, insight and sensation, is what's done at the insight barrier.

PART 2:

LITTLE EXPERIMENTS

I n Hakomi, we do little experiments as part of the work. Like, I noticed that with one woman, she had great difficulty looking me in the eyes. So, we did several experiments. I would close my eyes and she would notice what happened for her. Or, she would start by looking away and then slowly bring her eyes towards mine. We did several variations. Each time, she would be noticing what happened. She would tense or relax. She would have images and memories. All of that was gathering information about what core material organized this avoidance of eye contact. We did little experiments.

In all our techniques, there is an "experimental attitude." We study what's going on, not as disease or something to be rid of, but in an effort to help the client become conscious of how experience is managed and how the capacity for experience can be expanded. The whole endeavor is more fun and play rather than work and it is motivated by curiosity, rather than fear. This attitude recognizes the power of consciousness and places the healing forces in the client. In a relationship in which curiosity, mindfulness, self-direction and safety are key factors, honest and interesting questions can be asked and answered. Keeping to such an attitude is one of the tasks of the therapist. It is a way of putting some distance between the client and the therapist and also between the client and his or her "problem." It also tends to lessen the problems of transference. By studying, rather than fixing, we move away from the inevitability of unconsciously organized experience. We cultivate a healthy distance from the automatic and habitual, learning to use them wisely rather than feeling used by them.

Doing little experiments when interesting things come up in therapy changes the flavor completely. There's no emergency. Everything is "grist for the mill." The client has this or that to report and is very likely stuck in it, blind to what's going on and wants the therapist to change something. On the other hand, there must be something in the client doesn't want to change, or it would have just happened. When the therapist takes the attitude that this is something we can study, it shifts the central activity from doing to learning, the approach from avoiding to acknowledging. A slower, quieter pace is possible. Little experiments are ways the therapist keeps therapy from being problem solving, from being sturm and drang, from a litany of complaints and focused on suffering. It turns the enterprise into one of growth and self-knowledge. That in itself is therapeutic.

Probes and taking over are specific kinds of little experiments. We ask, "what happens when... " and then we do something. Other kinds of experiments have to do with the client noticing what happens when the therapist does something like walk away or towards the client slowly. Or, when the client tries to talk slowly, or studies a smile that appears at what seems are inappropriate times. Almost anything can be turned into something to experiment with. But it must be done without making the client feel disregarded or that he or she is being treated like an object. The relationship must be strong enough. The cooperation must be there. In that context, experimenting works.

Growth

Some people will question how can we promote growth when we are being so supportive and not frustrating dependencies. They believe that if you don't frustrate the client's attempts to elicit support, the client won't learn to use his own resources. In Hakomi Therapy, the very things we take over are the client's attempts at self-support and self-control, things the client is already doing for himself. We take over the client's habitual self-supporting, like the tensions that help manage the flow of feeling.

These are not things the client is asking us to do or trying to manipulate us into doing. These are the very areas in which the client's beliefs would show that no support is possible. We're offering support in areas in which the client does not ask questions and has no expectations, areas in which the client collapses into managing needs, wants and pain in ways that minimize experience and limit growth. By offering this support, we give the client new strength and new resources to go beyond merely managing pain and frustration to reorganizing and expanding.

In Hakomi Therapy, the object is to contact and work with core material. We foster growth by making it as safe and as easy as possible to bring core material to consciousness in order to change the influence of that material on the organization of experience. There are two ways, at least, to promote personal growth. One is to frustrate dependencies and the other is to directly support efforts toward growth. At one stage, the mother nurses the young and lets them be dependent. At another stage, she weans them and teaches them ways to get their own food. It is the combination of frustrating one thing and supporting another that helps direct the path of growth.

By taking something over, while staying with the experience, we are (1) offering support for the client's efforts to manage experience, to control the flow of feelings and images, to feel safe and understandable, while (2) simultaneously encouraging conscious, direct experience of those painful memories, feelings and beliefs that have so far gone unexamined.

If we frustrate anything at all it's the impulse to cover up and ignore what's going on at the level of core material, to just sit and talk and drift about, without looking seriously at one's own inner world. But I must say there's very little frustration or dependency that I've noticed. I believe that's simply because the impulse to personal freedom, power and self-reliance is, in the long run, always the stronger impulse. By supporting mindfulness and the effort to understand, we promote growth.

9

ACCESSING, DEEPENING, AND THE TRANSITION TO PROCESSING

PART 1:

ACCESSING

This section covers the principles and techniques of accessing. The term is borrowed from the computer sciences and is used to describe operations that make information available. Gaining access is the process that unlocks the path to information not otherwise available. For us, that often means taking the client from one state of consciousness into another. We use accessing techniques to help the client go from ordinary consciousness to mindfulness or from either one of those states to the child state. During mindfulness, we deepen the therapy process by accessing core material. In these ways, accessing is part of the transition to processing states.

In psychotherapy, the information we want is the beliefs, habits and memories that motivate and organize the client's reactions — the core material. This information is not ordinarily in consciousness or even available to it. The core helps organize the contents of consciousness while remaining outside. In the case of painful material, it may be kept outside of consciousness by strong habits. Still, it is this information that shapes our emotional life and gives it meaning. It has symbolic as well as emotional impact. It names our experiences and determines how we use the basic elements of our existence.

Such information has been called by many names. Karl Popper calls it intuitive belief[1]. Joseph Campbell's "mythic images" is another phrase[2]. I like both terms. "Intuitive beliefs" suggests the non-verbal, non-objectified state of this information. It is intuitive, non-verbal; it is felt or sensed, rather than thought. Yet, at the same time, it is acted on; it guides actions. So, truly, it is belief. Acted upon, yet not verbal, it may be stored as images and memories, which strongly suggests a right brain origin. These images organize experience. They summarize events, feelings, relationships, and decisions. They structure varied combinations of attitudes sensed in others and ourselves and the habits we react to them with. They are summarized, symbolized, compact and mysterious, like pictures in a dream.

We want access to the deepest intuitive beliefs, the most powerful behavior motivators, the "myths we live by," the personal myths, that are not consciously recognized most of the time. With more or less difficulty, they are available to consciousness but they haven't yet been examined mindfully. They haven't been clearly verbalized and so can't be questioned or doubted. When they are unavailable for doubt, they are also unavailable for change. It is only words that can be doubted and that is why these beliefs must be brought into consciousness and verbalized. Without that, they do not change[3]. In some cases, as I've said, they are painful and systematically avoided. For instance, the habit of tightening certain muscles in response to a thought usually happens outside of awareness. A therapist can bring that muscle tension into awareness just by mentioning it. What is more difficult is to bring into awareness those memories and beliefs that first created and now sustain the tension habit. And that's the information we want access to.

There's no way to get that information during ordinary consciousness. There's no talking to the driver while the bus is in motion. You can't take the engine apart while it's running. Any information that controls a particular operation is not available for change while the operation is in progress. This is a rule in computer operation and it is true for human operation as well. It wouldn't work - we wouldn't work - any other way. That's why we need mindfulness, a state of consciousness where all our "operations" are suspended. In mindfulness, we're not doing anything. Just like the wonder of childhood that's open and not doing anything in particular. ("Where did you go?" "Out." "What did you do?" "Nothing.") That kid-like "nothing" makes the inner world available.

You can't access people while they're busy. The busy mind won't let you access its belief systems. The busy mind is not taking incoming calls. That's how my old friend Junior Peacock used to describe the drugged state: "no incoming calls." The busy mind is using those beliefs to operate with. It's dangerous to go ahead and try to change them while you're in the middle of some thing. No time to take the ladder apart when you're up two floors and standing on it. Your belief systems are protected when you're busy. They are protected from interruption when your awareness is focused outside yourself, when you are concerned about ongoing, external matters, when you're goal directed. To access information about character, we must give up behaving characteristically, at least for the moment.

Such information is available only in special states of consciousness. We all know the quality of these special states. We've all experienced them. Sitting and gazing... the wonder of childhood... we know those. In these states, belief systems are available in a very special way and not just to the logical mind. No, they are not just matters for discussion. States of consciousness like wonder and mindfulness are not intellectual states at all. They are states in which our contact with pure experience is very strong. Our organizing beliefs are very real for us then, and that's when they are available: when they are felt as real, when they are felt reality. Indeed, Eugene Gendlin uses the term "felt sense"[4].

Organizing beliefs don't arise simply as philosophical possibilities. They come with conviction and all the emotional charge that created them. People don't just say with calm, casual voices, "Nobody ever loved me." If that is a real part of your beliefs, it won't manifest so mildly. It will arrive with grief too heavy to bear. Felt reality. Don't confuse discussing reality with accessing a belief system!

There are lots of ways to get into these altered states of consciousness, through ritual dancing, yoga, hypnosis, poetry, art, mythology, music, drugs, and so on. Rituals, ceremonies, meditation, all these are ways to access. They are ways to focus on internal signals while lowering the noise. If you want to help people change on a deep level, you must first help them enter one of these special states. You must help them access. Once they have accessed they can go ahead and process whatever it is that has come up. They can, if they're mindful, also notice how they are being affected by what comes up. They can observe it all happening. We've been calling that mindfulness and "witnessing." There are certain, specific operations in Hakomi Therapy that access, that bring about mindfulness and create the witness.

Perls accessed by asking people to stay in the here and now, and then pointed out things that were going on just outside of their awareness[5]. He kept them in a little bit of a trance. Or, you can think of it as a little bit out of the ego-trance we're usually in. Milton Erickson's accessing techniques were practically miraculous[6]. Gendlin has a very simple accessing technique that's quite effective. He calls it "focusing," and he wrote about it in a book by the same name. The accessing techniques I use have the qualities of maintaining conscious awareness and memory and proceeding always within the boundaries of permission and choice on the part of the client. These qualities are consistent with the principles of mindfulness and nonviolence and continue to guide the process before and after accessing takes place.

Guidelines for Accessing

The following four guiding principles are associated with accessing. If you practice them till they become habit, you'll have no trouble accessing:

Safety. First, create a safe situation. You have to create, or help create, a feeling of security in the persons you're working with. If they don't feel safe, they won't drop external awareness; they won't trust the outside world enough to go inside. If they don't feel safe, they'll be watching you, keeping an eye on you. You, personally, have to be a safe place for the client. They must feel safe enough to relinquish purpose, time and consciousness of their surroundings in order to go inside themselves. Whenever there's trouble accessing, I try to find out what will make a person feel safer. "Is there anything that would make you feel more comfortable?" That kind of question. Let the person work on getting more comfortable. Sometimes a client wants to know that you're not going to do this or that. Making the person safe is the first order of business.

The therapist must be totally committed to protecting the feelings and spirit of the client. That means the therapist puts plans and judgments and "success" second to protecting the spirit. You may have some qualities about you that threaten this person. You'd better deal with that. What's making them uncomfortable? For example, needing to get some kind of response from them. Having a plan in mind for them. Judging them. These things can be very subtle and they create insecurities in the client. The best thing you can do is to be totally accepting. If you can be loving, accepting and nonjudgmental, the person is most likely going to feel safe. You have to have a commitment to protect the person's spirit. I get angry and disgusted at those therapy techniques that insult people and deliberately create pain. There's already plenty of pain to handle. And God knows our spirits have been insulted! If you are skillful, you can coax pain from its hiding places and offer some relief. There's no need to create any more of it.

Also, you must be "congruent" (Carl Rogers' term). Don't say things you don't mean. People can pick that up and, again, the situation will not be safe. They won't know what to believe. They'll have to watch you. If your voice is angry, though your words be sweet as candy, you won't access anyone. And remember, it's people's beliefs that actually determine when they're comfortable. And we're trying to access those same beliefs. It won't help to reason with them. Just do what you must to make them more comfortable. Avoiding confrontation and being "on their side" is more important than being right about anything.

Present Experience. The second guideline of accessing is this: help the clients to focus on and to stay with their present experience. What you're trying to access are the core material and support structures behind organized experience. You want the person to experience that material as felt reality, not as theory. Felt reality is feelings, moods, thoughts, and muscle tension that are happening right now. You want the clients to "know" their beliefs in this live sense, not just in the idea sense. You want to bring them to the felt sense of this present moment. That's when it's possible to change it. You can't change direction until you come to that particular crossroad.

In over 90% of the cases in which therapy doesn't work, it's because accessing hasn't happened. Gendlin has shown that if the client doesn't stay with his or her experience, therapy doesn't happen. Gendlin trained students to listen to the tapes of the first and second sessions of ongoing psychotherapy and they could predict with better than 90% accuracy which therapist/client combinations were going to work and which weren't. They could tell from the first two sessions. You could probably do it in the first fifteen minutes in many cases. And the simple reason for therapy not working is this: the clients did not stay with present experience. The therapist asks for a report on something that's happening and doesn't get experience. The therapist asks the client about feelings, and the client replies, "Well, I don't know what that was," or offers only reasons and explanations. You ask what's going on now and the client starts talking about last Thursday at the A & P. As far as experience goes, that's upping the noise. That's when therapy doesn't happen. You ask the person for experience and you get noise.

I find this the most difficult principle for people to get early in training. I think it's because this constraint is not used anywhere else. The habits of following another person's tendency to talk of the past, to conjecture and theorize, and so on, following what's interesting, being polite, these habits of ordinary conversation are very strong. Don't get hooked on stories about the past. Don't get hooked on drama. Come right back to the present. Ask for concrete experience. Ask questions that can only be answered if the person stays with present experience. You have to ask only two or three of these kinds of questions in a row before the person is stabilized in the present. After you've accessed, the person automatically stays with his or her experience.

One way is to ask for precise information about something that's going on now. For example, if somebody says he's sad, don't ask what the sadness is about! That's the royal road to explanation. Ask, "what kind of sadness is it!" Then the client goes right back into the sadness. Deeper. The sadness becomes much more informative. With that search comes memories and, finally, beliefs. At almost any moment, the therapist can ask a question which will redirect the client towards present experience. It may not follow logically but, if the client is cooperating, it will lead to accessing. You will be a psychological Aikido master when you can take anything a person says or does and turn it towards present experience.

Slowly. Another guideline is: go slowly! If you're going fast, clients can only react. They'll do that to keep pace with you. We don't want reactions, we want experience and mindfulness. Reactions happen at one speed, awareness at another. The various states of consciousness operate differently in time. To examine the way behavior is organized, you have to slow down. The neurons that mediate awareness are more complexly connected and far slower than those that mediate consciousness. If you learned long ago to play a piece of music very well on a piano and somebody asks you now how you finger it, you can't sit there and remember that. You've got to slow down and actually notice how you've organized that particular experience.

For example, from what we know about neurophysiology, when Isaac Stern plays a very fast piece on his violin, he can't be "thinking" one finger at a time. He's got to send down messages which move his fingers in set sequences. He sends down whole blocks of information about movements to his fingers. The brain cannot move one finger, notice it, and then move another fast enough to get down the arm and back, and still account for playing as fast as Isaac Stern is able to play. So that information comes down in chunks. When you're going fast, information is chunked. To experience, to notice and to understand exactly the details of your movements, you've got to unchunk then. You have to slow down. When you're accessing, you must go slowly. You must give the client time. You are evoking mindfulness. When you go slowly, you are inviting the client to go slowly. You are inviting self-observation. Similarly, when you ask for information, you have to ask in such a way that you are acknowledging that there is plenty of time. Speech that accesses is different from normal speech. The tone of voice, the speed at which you talk, the gentleness with which you move, all of this says "you're safe," "take your time," "go inward." In all non-ordinary states—hypnosis, for example—the form and timing of the communication are essential to accessing.

Nonviolence. Finally, the fourth guideline: go gently! You must be nonviolent. Nonviolence and mindfulness are the pillars of Buddhism, the way to knowledge of the higher self. In working with others: always kindness, always compassion! Never work against anyone's will or wishes! You must avoid setting off the defense systems. You want to "come in under the radar." If you are violent, you disturb the others, and they leave their inner experience and turn outward to deal with you. Remember, there are many levels of violence! Judgments, plans, advice, exclusion of any kind, and the arrogance that many therapists show, all are violent and each creates defenses in the other person. But inclusion, empowerment and nonviolence give others the room to do what they will and to be who they are, without any need to change that. Accessing needs the presence of this kind of acceptance and support.

During this entire accessing process, you should be tracking the signals which tell you which way this person's process wants to go and you should be making contact. You're constantly sending them signals that you're following their experience. As soon as clients know you're with them and are going to help them to do what they want to do, they access easily.

So, note these four: creating safety, asking for experience, going slowly, and being gentle — the four guidelines of accessing. They create the delicate mixture which allows the opening to the sources of the self.

PART 2:

DEEPENING

A
ccessing brings the client into a state of mindfulness. Once that happens, our object is to stabilize that state and deepen it first and then to use it to access core material. In mindfulness the process moves readily towards those beliefs, memories, and so on which most need to come forth. A relaxation of control and a feeling of safety allow the unconscious to yield material normally kept out of awareness. The client and therapist are engaged not only in a conscious dialogue, but very much in an unconscious one as well. At this early point the therapist begins to understand where the process is going. The meaning of what's happening begins to become clear. Still, it behooves the therapist to go slowly now, to deepen and stabilize mindfulness before going for core material.

When mindfulness arrives, it comes in response to the therapist's instructions to the client simply to... "be aware of what happens... when I..." or "when you..." and then doing a probe or taking something over or instructing the client to do something. The first time, the therapist may also explain what is wanted: a turning inward to observe what happens, without needing to do anything. The signs of mindfulness, slowness and softness of speech, patient concentration, reports on present experience, should all be showing. Deepening and stabilizing this state is a simple matter.

We ask questions about the present experience that require the client to stay in the experience to answer the questions. We ask questions that require more precise answers. If the reaction to a probe say was "My face tingled," then a deepening question might be, "Is your face tingling more on the right side or the left?" An important point about such questions is that the therapist may not need or even want the information they yield. The therapist may not be the least interested in which side of the face tingles more or whatever. It is just a technique for deepening and stabilizing mindfulness. Two or three questions like that and the client generally settles down and remains mindful without further ado. It's useful to make contact statements during the deepening process. Contact helps set up the rhythm of the interaction just as it would in a normal conversation.

Occasionally, the therapist will have to instruct clients, particularly those with expressive or industrious processes, to stay inside. Certain people have a pattern of doing a task and then coming to you to report about it as something from the immediate past. Such a habit could keep the therapy from going anywhere at all. Like a game of ping-pong, the client goes back and forth from mindfulness to reporting in ordinary consciousness, while the therapist goes from task to task. It's a pattern that inexperienced therapists often fall into. To stop that should it start happening, instruct such clients to stay with their experience and report about it in the present tense, while it's happening, without opening their eyes and without coming out of the mind-attention state. It may take a time or two to get it, but most clients can and will.

In deepening, some clients will at first be mindful only of what may seem trivialities. The client may report, say, in response to a probe, "My wrist started itching." Some people, first report mostly sensations. It is a simple matter to ask deepening questions about those sensations and, at a point not too much later, the client will begin to report feelings - often quite suddenly. The overall shift in the course of deepening is from (1) thoughts and ideas, to (2) images, sensations and tensions, to (3) feelings, and finally to (4) whole memories, experiences and in sights. The overall shift is also from local sensations, tensions, feelings, etc., to more global, whole body events.

Riding the rapids could start at any time. When it does, the pursuit of mindfulness is temporarily abandoned and the techniques appropriate to the rapids are used. Some clients will not be able to stay in mindfulness at all. Usually, they are just too tense, anxious or nervous. If you've done everything you can to access and deepen mindfulness and it doesn't work, then discuss safety issues and try to find a way to reduce the tension, like an energetic, physical interaction. If that doesn't work, the client needs some other approach, like massage, a change in diet, a vacation, or what have you. They're not ready for Hakomi Therapy or it's not ready for them and that fact has to be faced directly, albeit delicately.

Of course, some clients will experience and report feelings and memories almost immediately and others will be able to access and stabilize mindfulness very quickly. Once mindfulness is accessed and stabilized, the task is to access core material.

PART 3:

THE TRANSITION TO PROCESSING

W hen the client is deeply involved, mindful and taking time with questions and reports, the whole process takes on its own pace. There's a live quality to it, energizing and engaging. By now, the therapist has developed some notions about what kind of process it is and what kind of probe or technique will work to bring the client into contact with core material. A simple probe, at such times, can be all that's needed to bring on a deep, powerful experience for the client. At another time the same words might have little or no effect, but in mindfulness, at a time when the client is open, calm and attentive to reactions, the right words are like a key that suddenly opens the way to the client's very core.

An example: A client reports feelings of anger at the probe, "your life belongs to you." The client also feels a tightening of the abdominals. So, you or your assistant take over that tightening and put some pressure on the abdominals to simulate the tension. Now you try the probe again, with the client letting you take over the tension in the abdominals, and now the reaction is an explosion of feeling and a clear memory filled with rage and humiliation.

Or: The client senses a whole pattern of tension and you ask some questions to deepen the experience. The client tells you all about the sensations in this part and that, but always with the careful observations of mindfulness. Then, when you think it's time, you ask, "What does your body seem to be saying with that pattern of tensions?" We often attempt to access core material by going for the meaning of some bodily event. A bodily event that happens in reaction to a probe is, after all, part of a whole system of reactions, all organized and controlled by core beliefs, memories and so on. That intimate connection between reaction and core is what we use to access that material. The client realizes suddenly his body is saying, "touch me!" And with that, the feelings and the memories that make sense of that painful cry come forth.

In accessing core material, we go from present experience, sensations, feelings, thoughts, and so on, to beliefs, memories and images that, though they operate strongly and constantly on the present, are more a part of the hidden, painful past. We go from experience to the symbolic material that shapes all experience. Symbolic material has meaning beyond its simply having happened. Not only were the events powerful; they significantly influenced the way the person defined him or herself, important others and the world.

There is more to do, of course, though just getting to core material can be a powerful event in a person's life. This is deep, formative material, at the center of who the client is and how he or she came to be that. To be in contact with these old events is to seem to arrive home, to know oneself in the most real and significant way. It is to feel and know the almost holy power to choose who one will be. Not that it will be easy to change. There are strong reasons why we are the way we are. The forces that have shaped us will not trip lightly from the scene.

When core material comes up, it often brings with it a further shift in consciousness to those states we are calling, strong emotions or the child. These are specific states and the processing we do in them is specific also. In the chapters to follow, we discuss: working with the child, working with strong emotions, and going for meaning.

Notes for Chapter 9.

1. *The Self and Its Brain*, by Karl Popper and John Eccles
2. *Myths We Live By* and *Mythic Images*, by Joseph Campbell
3. The *Journal of Energy and Character*, by David Boadella
4. *Focusing*, by Eugene Gendlin
5. *Gestalt Therapy*, by Perls, Hefferline and Goodman
6. *Hypnotic Realities*, by Milton K. Erickson

10

WORKING WITH STRONG EMOTIONS: RIDING THE RAPIDS

As in any therapy that deals with deeply held beliefs and painful memories, strong feelings and the need to express those feelings arise. With safety and support established, the client may experience a spontaneous emotional release, possibly for the first time since childhood. Emotional release, once begun, becomes almost an organic need. It rushes out and, if it is not interrupted, flows to completion. The ability to work with emotions is an important part of the therapist's skills. Feelings are part of the biological foundations of behavior. They have a natural unfolding. The therapist's most important task during emotional release is to aid that unfolding, to support it and make it safe.

Since feeling is so important in therapy, some therapists deliberately promote its expression even in the face of resistance. In Hakomi we don't push through resistance, we process feelings when they arise spontaneously, without forcing them in any way. When emotional release is seen as central and the therapist deliberately promotes it, the resistance to emotions is thought of as a negative part of the client. A struggle often ensues in which the therapist and one part of the client attempt to experience and express feelings, while another part of the client habitually fights back. The effect is often conflict for the client, with feelings of guilt and failure on one side and a natural resistance to being forced on the other. The part that doesn't want to feel or express has a story too. We listen to it. When a way is found to acknowledge and accommodate both expression and control, the work with emotions is more integrated, less overwhelming and meets with little resistance.

All through the therapeutic process, we carefully track for the small signs that emotions are near and ready for release. At those times, we support the process of release. We do not provoke the client or try to exhaust the defenses in any way. We help manage the flow of feelings when they happen, by making them as safe as possible and letting them take their own course. By avoiding the confrontations, by being less insistent and less directive, we avoid arousing the defenses. By supporting the spontaneous aspects of emotional release, especially the tensions and postures the client habitually uses to manage strong feelings (the very things that are called resistance), we make the process safer and easier for the client to enter into. In my experience, this approach is more satisfying. An important goal of this approach is to bring mindfulness to the way we organize our experience. We want to study and understand the way we create the world in which we live. A serious study of that requires quiet, bare attention and a mind unfettered by strong feelings. Processing feelings helps clear the way for mindfulness. Still, feelings are a natural, important part of any life. They give substance and direction to experience. Finding ways to make them safe and satisfying is therapeutic in itself. So, we try to help our clients learn that their feelings are okay and that they can express those feelings with safe and satisfying results.

I think of the spontaneous expression of strong emotions as a specific state of consciousness. It is characterized by intense involvement, centered on present experience, spontaneous physical activity and limited capacity to think or reason. A great deal of energy is released. Explosions of rage, deep sobbing, the overwhelming pain of loss, feelings like these can fill the mind to overflowing. In therapy, such feelings tend to come in waves, with memories and insights bobbing between the crests. They seem uncontrollable, though much is going on to control them. In the struggle to control them, they become even more painful. Once the feelings are accepted as natural and okay, once they can be freely expressed and allowed to run their course, they are not only bearable, they are a relief. They may even feel pleasurable and wanted, as righteous anger can be or the grief that is a final loving message to the dead.

This state of consciousness is incompatible with mindfulness. The rapids are no place for studying. With white water all around and much to do to keep oneself afloat - it's no time for taking in the scenery. When a client goes into emotional processing, we do not ask for mindfulness. We drop the whole business of processing in mindfulness, searching for meaning, probes and so on, and do only a few simple things like holding the person and offering some contact or nourishing statements. There's not much conversation and few, if any, questions. Any dialogue is done on the level of movement and physical contact as the therapist moves to help the client with tensions and expression. For that, very little talk is necessary. But, spontaneous movements and changes in posture do happen. Muscles tense involuntarily. This is the natural result of the client's use of automatic habits to manage intense feelings. They are emergency procedures, for what we have here is emergence. Since these habits have been for the most part out of awareness, they are surprising to the client and seem to have a life of their own. We are in areas of the client's life that have not been dealt with in this way before.

The most important task the therapist has during emotional release is: support spontaneous behavior! The spontaneous movements and tensions, even the gestures clients make in this state, are all ways the client is managing his or her experience. That management is mostly unconscious and closely tied to core material. Anything we do to support it is recognized on the deepest levels as such. We create safety and are allowed to participate in these levels of the client's process. Opposition to the spontaneous separates us from the other and makes us part of the problem. So, we support the spontaneous.

Of course, to do that, you have to know what spontaneous behavior looks and sounds like. You have to be able to differentiate between feelings being forced and feelings that can't be stopped. Some people can "produce" intense expressions at will. They usually do so in the service of an expressive/clinging strategy. These people can take a small feeling or a seemingly unemotional event and turn it into a full-blown experience. It is dramatized. That doesn't mean it's not important. It is. But what's important isn't what the drama is about, but the need to dramatize itself. At times like those, when you're getting drama, there are ways to work which do not focus on supporting spontaneous behavior. For now its enough to know that the expression of strong feeling isn't always spontaneous.

Forced feelings sound forced; they lack authenticity and naturalness. They sound dramatic. As you work with someone who is forcing feelings, and you haven't noticed the forcing, it's likely that you yourself will eventually start feeling something. If you're trying to get something to happen, you'll become frustrated. If you're just following the process, you'll start to get bored. Not because it isn't feelingful; it's that and more. But, the feelings are all in the service of something else, the continuance of the relationship. So, no matter how much you try to help the person feel better, something new to have strong feelings about will always arise. The whole process doesn't seem to be going anywhere. It won't until you address the real issue: the need to dramatize. So, your own experience can tell you that the process isn't spontaneous.

When feelings are spontaneous, the situation moves. It unfolds. Clients can be very emotional, surprised, overwhelmed. Still, they let you participate. They want and accept support. They're being real and it shows in the way they look at you and respond to you. Oddly enough, the person with spontaneous feelings will be struggling with them much more than will the person who is forcing. In the spontaneous process, there's real resistance. There is spontaneous, automatic tensions and movements that you just don't see any other time. These are the signs that tell you how to support the process. You support the process by taking over as much of the tension as possible. For example, if the person you're working with contracts inward, hugging themselves and closing down, folding up, you move to help them do that. You put your arms around them, from the back even, and you help them contract. You hold them tight as you would a child who is tense and frightened. When you do that, the person's body may relax a little. This can happen without your saying anything. With support given and felt at the deepest levels, the control relaxes and the process moves on. The unconscious feels its opportunities and takes them.

If the head turns to one side as they are lying on the floor, possibly crying, you help turn them, taking the whole body and, gently, with their permission, rolling them on their side. Turning and folding are spontaneous ways we protect ourselves at these times. All sorts of contractions and tensions are used to ease the flow of feelings. Covering the eyes happens a lot. Tightness in the abdomen is another. By taking these things over, you help the process along. All these spontaneous actions are ways the client defends against too much feeling. By helping with this managing and defending, you acknowledge, without judgment, the very real experience the client is having. That, too, helps the process along. It is like a physical contact statement. It says, "I know what's happening and I accept it. I'm willing to help you do whatever you feel you have to do." It says, "I'm patient. I'm following what's happening. I'm here with you and its your process." Those are things the client wants to know.

Following are some additional situations you'll typically have to take over and support:

1. The lower spine may rise up off the floor. Put a hand under it, taking the weight of the lower back. Do the same for the back of the neck.
2. If the knees come up, support them in that position.
3. If the shoulders come up off the floor while the person is on his or her back, take them over as well.
4. Look for little bits of tension, for example, in the toes or the fore head, etc., which can be taken over, too.
5. The hands cover the eyes or the whole face, indicating an impulse to hide. Gently place your own hands over the client's face, or offer to use your hands in place of theirs.

In many cases, the client will go in and out of the rapids, alternating strong expression with moments of clarity and relative calm. Islands in the stream. At those times of calm, which can last as long as several minutes, the therapist can talk to the child or the unconscious, can make contact statements and perhaps ask a few questions. But even then, the focus is on making it safe; the search for nourishment and understanding is secondary. This state of consciousness is totally new for some people and rare for most. A person going through such an experience may feel out of control or even crazy. It is the calm, reassuring demeanor of the therapist which silently and most effectively says, "You're all right. What is going on here is perfectly natural and, as intense as it is, it's understandable and nothing to worry about." It pays to convey that message. As therapists, we are part of some of the most intimate and powerful experiences people have. Our use to those people is partly in our ability to stay calm and compassionate throughout.

When people are emotional, they're also open and susceptible. It's both an opportunity and a time to be careful. The opportunity is that it's a good time to make nourishing statements. You can simply offer the statements without asking for mindfulness or reports. You can offer several, one after the other. It helps, of course, if you've been paying attention all along and have a good idea of what's going to be nourishing. At such times it is wise to avoid saying anything with negative implications. The person is open and vulnerable. A statement with negative implications could be accepted uncriticaly, perhaps even go unnoticed. So, let's be careful out there!

When Nothing Works

I'll tell you what happens when all the stuff I'm trying doesn't work? The person is riding the rapids and I'm trying to support spontaneous behavior, or I'm trying to offer nourishment, or I ask the person about what's going on and I don't get an answer. No response! At that point, I go back to making contact. If I'm not getting responses from the person when I ask for reports, I'll make a contact statement like, "difficult to talk now, huh." In response the person may nod or something. So, I'll try to come back into contact. That's item one. I may also simply report what I imagine the person is experiencing. Very often the person just can't talk at the moment. The feelings are too strong.

So, I try to come back into contact. If you're constantly supporting spontaneous behavior, you don't need any answers. It's only when the person seems stuck that you need to do some thing about it. If the process is going along fine, without words, that's okay. You're contacting, offering nourishing statements, naming a belief or two. That's fine. It's when the process seems to be stuck, grinding away, when the person seems to be pushing, then you have to do something about it. It's not just the expressive/clinging process that gets stuck. The industrious/ over focused process gets stuck too. The client gets onto something and starts pushing, trying, stifling the spontaneous. I will interrupt the pushing and take a break or try something else or focus on the pushing itself.

After the ride, if the client signals a readiness for it, I go for meaning, by clarifying beliefs, or going back to mindfulness and working with probes again.

The relaxation that follows emotional release creates a quieting of the system, a lowering of the noise. This quietness provides a rich opportunity for accessing more subtle signals (feelings, sensations, needs, images). So it is a good time to work on integration or meaning. If a new experience has been gained, that is a transformation has taken place, I support the client's efforts to integrate. Sometimes though, the person has had enough for now and lets me know he feels that way. Then, I just let the person rest comfortably, maybe staying there to hold him and listen to him while we both get a little rest.

11

WORKING WITH THE CHILD: THE THERAPIST AS MAGICAL STRANGER

The experiences we evoke in therapy often relate directly to early childhood. In evoking these, we often evoke along with them, something of the child who had them. It occurs as a spontaneous shift in consciousness and it emerges under the influence of emotionally charged memories. In remembering the feelings and events of childhood, we remember also the consciousness of childhood. It involves another non-ordinary state of consciousness, the child state. (Its special properties are discussed below.) If we take notice and respond to this special state, we can talk and interact directly with the child who, in his consciousness, is still in the situation that shaped his life. We call that working with the child.

Things learned in one state of consciousness may be quite difficult to access from another state of consciousness. Remembering dreams is one example. Hypnosis is another. When you hypnotize a well trained subject by having him count down from one hundred, (100 ...99 ...98 ...97 ...96 ...etc.) the subject can go into trance after only seven or eight numbers. Once in trance, you can take the hypnotized person outside, walk him around, and do whatever activities you like. As long as the subject stays in the hypnotic state, you can spend hours that way. Then, if you go back to the place where you first hypnotized the person — the same room, chair, lighting, and physical posture — you can bring the subject out of trance simply by asking the subject to wake up. The subject often picks up the count exactly where he left off, many hours earlier, (94... 93.... 92...). The person won't know for a while that several hours have gone by.

That's a wonderful example of state-specific memory. The count that eight hours ago begins the moment the subject starts to come out of the hypnotic state and back into ordinary consciousness. He simply continues where he left off. The point is, memory can be discontinuous with changes in states. Working with the child involves this state-specific memory. The child who had those early experiences was in a much different state of consciousness than the adult he or she became. So different, in fact, that most adults have great difficulty remembering what they were like as a child. Yet it was the child's experiences that created the core material that still influences all behavior.

The child state is quite different from the hypnotic state, however. The person in the child state of consciousness hasn't lost his connections to the real immediate situation. The child he was and the adult he is are present at the same time. So, it's not just the child that is present; the adult is here also. A client in the child state almost always knows exactly where he is. He knows he is sitting in your office. He knows you're a therapist, etc. His real adult life is still going on. At the same time, the person feels like a child, a very real, live child, vividly experiencing itself and its world. The state can be intense enough so the person is carried away with the emotions of the child and it can be delicate and easily lost, or anywhere in between. The client may be in touch with a particular event or experience lost or forgotten for many years. He may be seeing faces and hearing voices long forgotten. And it all comes back vividly, with clear images and thoughts the child had in the original situation. The client is again experiencing things the way the child did. These are not just imagined events; they are important pieces of unfinished business.

There's another significant thing about both the adult and the child being present: it's a great opportunity to do some integrating. It allows the client to relive some painful experience and to watch it at the same time. It is a great chance to understand one's history, combining the emotional intensity of childhood with the reasoning capabilities of an adult. In a way, it's the best of both worlds.

Children are shaped by events in ways that rarely affect adults because the child is still mostly unshaped. The child is open and still learning. The child is still creating the way it deals with the world. It's still learning to organize its experience. The life of the child is a life at the core. So, when we focus on the organization of experience, on character processes and core material, we're close to the realm of the child. If we know the signs, we can contact that child, bring that whole state of consciousness into operation and work with it directly.

When you evoke experiences in mindfulness, or deepen, or go for meaning, when you are working with character processes, you are quite likely to evoke the child. It's the child after all who first created and used the character strategies. When I first started doing psychotherapy, I never tried to get in contact with the child. I didn't know about it. As I gained experience, the child state began to appear spontaneously. Slowly, I learned to expect it, to notice it quickly, and I even developed some techniques for deliberately evoking it.

The child and its experiences built the world view and the self-image. The child was the map maker. So, in contacting and working with the child, you have the possibility of changing those maps and the person who is now using them. By working with that child. By just being there with that child, by talking to it and holding it and explaining things, by being careful and concerned and patient, just by doing that, you change the way that child feels about itself and the world. And in doing that, you change the adult, too.

The child can and does emerge quite naturally. The therapist can also help it to emerge. It can arise naturally in many ways. Sometimes an image appears in which the client sees himself as a child. Sometimes the client gets a feeling of being a child in a particular situation. Sometimes the child state comes complete with scenes and events right from the start and sometimes it begins slowly, with something sensory. Sometimes it just appears as part of the style of interaction with the therapist. The person gets childish. One man I was working with suddenly remembered the smell of cardboard. At that point, he was still in ordinary consciousness and only mildly curious. I asked him if it was wet cardboard or dry cardboard. He stayed with the experience and then, quite suddenly, he grew terrified and began to vividly re-experience being in a burning cardboard box. Some other children had put him in the box and had set it on fire.

At times I deliberately evoke the child. Once I asked a woman who had come from out-of-state to work with me, how she'd gotten here. She told me that she'd come by plane. As she answered, I noticed a little light in her eyes, so I asked her, with that special voice you might use with a child who might have something exciting to report, "Could you see out of the window?" Her manner took on a child's delight. She started telling me about all the things she saw looking out the window and got quickly into being a child again. Another time, there was a woman sitting in my waiting room when I arrived at the office. There was something in the way she was sitting and looking at me. I knew her, but I'd never worked with her before. I felt she was close to her child. I walked up to her, touched the tip of her nose and asked with that same special voice, "What's this?" She turned right into a three-year old and said with a sweet little pout, "That's my nose." As I took her hand and we went into my office, I was saying to the child, "You're unhappy about something, aren't you."

Sometimes the child emerges at a distance. It comes as an image of a child. A client may report seeing herself as a child or remembering herself as a child. The client may actually see the child a few feet away, doing something while the present adult watches. I think that indicates that the client isn't ready to actually experience the child. If that's the case, you can use the adult to talk to the child, to intervene with the child and report to you about what's happening. Sometimes I'll ask the person, "Can I talk to the child?" "Will you talk to the child for me?" "I'd like to talk to her; would you tell her this?" Something like that, using the adult as an intermediary. Sometimes that will evolve into the person being the child, and sometimes you just have to stay with the adult as intermediary. The person though not ready to actually re-experience being the child, may still be ready to deal with the issues.

When the image of the child appears at a distance, it may also be that the person doesn't want to own that child, or hates the child, hates that part of herself. It's important then to try to create a dialogue and eventual reunion with the child. I asked one woman to reach out and touch the child part she hated. She couldn't do it. She hated the child; she didn't want to touch it. She wanted it to go away, which means, stay buried. So, I had her try reaching out while I held her back. As we explored what she hated about the child, she realized, "She always got me in trouble. She was always being bad." She hated that part of herself for getting her in trouble. The reunion began when she remembered how painfully unloved that part of her felt. At the deepest levels, reconciliation is strongly wanted. Often such negative self-images dissolve as soon as the reunion happens. Hakomi trainer Pat Ogden worked with a woman who had an image of her infant self as a reptile, as hideous as it could be. When Pat had her reach out and touch it, it changed immediately to a baby that needed her love and attention.

Though the child may emerge only as an image at a distance, you can still be waiting for it. You can watch for and listen for the signs: a change in the voice, a flash of the child in the facial expression, a small gesture, childlike wording and sentences. The signs will often appear in response to a probe. I'll try a probe and, as the person reports his or her reaction, there's the faint echo of a child there. Quite often, it goes unnoticed by the client. The client doesn't know that he or she just went childish. I'll point it out somehow and do something to stabilize it. Like any other state of consciousness, the child state has to be deepened and stabilized. When I notice the child, I may ask about it. Sometimes I just ask, "How old do you feel now?" Mostly, I just contact the feeling or its presents. "Feeling young now, huh." Or, "so the child is here now, huh."

Once, I asked this of a woman whose voice had just become childish and at first she wasn't aware of it. When I asked her how old she felt, she answered, "My usual age." I asked, "How old is that?" At that point she started to hear and feel herself. She was going to say, "thirty-two" and stopped for a moment, then continued with, "well, maybe I'm three." The child came through easily and we touched on how very much she wanted to be loved by her father but felt she wasn't. We worked on that for a while and finally got to a place where she could imagine having a father who loved her. To integrate the feeling of being loved, I helped her re-live out her whole life in fantasy, with this new, loving father. She told me what happened when she first went to school, what he did when she graduated from high school, etc. It took about forty-five minutes. When she got to be 32 again, her life was totally different. She had a different profession, different attitudes on health. The contrast between the result of her imagined life and her regular life was amazing.

In working with the child, the first thing to do is to make contact. Basically it's done by shifting your manner and tone of voice. You just start talking as if you were talking to a child. (One of the reasons it's good to do probes in very simple language is that doing so evokes the child.) You can ask what's happening or how old the person feels. Usually, they will find a precise age for you. In the process of finding the exact age, the experience deepens. Contact statements also work. Mostly it's contact statements and using your voice as if you were talking to a child. Another way to deepen the state is to get more detail about the event or the situation the child is in. If an image emerges, like "Ah, I can see the bars of my crib," you say, "Well, look down now, what color blanket do you have? What else do you see in the room?" Just keep them in the experience long enough to stabilize it. Or, you can ask, "What do people call you?" And, if they spoke a different language at that time, you can ask them to say a few words in that language. Sometimes that's very significant. Just tell them to speak in their original language. You don't have to know what it means. There are enough other clues to what's going on and you can find out later.

After we've accessed the child, we work with her or him. What do we do with the child once it is there and the state is stable? I have already talked about working through the adult, getting the adult to take care of the child, getting the adult to talk to the child. Because I'm such a tough/generous guy, I like to appear as a magical stranger. Other people assume different personal styles as magical stranger. I like to talk to the child and demonstrate that I understand it. I like to help it understand what's going on in its world and to help it with its concept of itself. If the child feels that something unjust has just happened, it could also get the idea that the world is always unjust and that it will never get fair treatment. I just talk a while about that, how maybe people could treat the child better, more fairly and that even though it happened maybe a lot to them, it doesn't always have to be that way. I may also elicit from the child, its sense of what is right and fair. Basically, I just talk to the child as if I had come upon it at that very moment in its life. And I do what you can, as any intelligent, compassionate adult would who had come upon that child in that situation.

I call that role I'm taking on, the magical stranger. Magical, because you appear in the original situation, where you never really were. And stranger, because I'm not there as anybody else, just me. I'm not the child's father or uncle or anyone they already know. I focus on understanding and on absorbing and integrating these events. The situation was traumatic and is back now, because it didn't resolve then. It was too painful or too confusing. The child was overwhelmed. So I help the child to understand. I just talk like an adult, with adult experience. I'm sympathetic and I go at the child's pace. But I don't try to change history or paint rosy pictures. I just offer my honest, humanly limited understanding for the child to consider and contact the child's feelings and vision of the events. I'm also good at guessing what happened and that helps the child to accept and believe in me. So, I focus on understanding while at the same time, supporting the child emotionally. Very often I'm touching the person, holding them, wiping the tears away, doing small, natural adult-and-child things. I hold the kleenex and have the client blow his nose. Little things like that.

I focus on what the child needs (or needed) in that situation. It needed somebody to come along and do something, to tell it about death or whatever. To make sense of what the adults were doing. I let the child's needs guide the process. But that, of course, is what we always do.

If the child is preverbal, I use a lot of contact statements. Preverbal states are more difficult. A lot of good tracking of the body is necessary. A typical thing is a situation where the person re-experiences birth. The person feels like they want to push with their legs, so I support those movements. I provide them some kind of confinement and hold them while they stay with their breathing. I let them open their eyes slowly and see someone friendly and loving. Sometimes I do the work with no words at all. When they are afraid to open their eyes, I have an assistant report everything that is going on in the visual field while the client leaves his or her eyes closed. We take over seeing.

As part of my work with the child, as I help the child understand, one thing I try to do is make the parents real and understandable. The child's experience of his or her parents is almost surely mixed with uncertainties and distortions. It is a great relief to have those cleared up and resolved. I discuss with the child how the parents feel (or felt), how they have pain and confusion of their own, how they may have tried to do what they thought was best for the child. This isn't an apology for the parents; it's just to bring them down to size and show they were simply human. I work with the fact that as an adult, the person doesn't need his or her parents the same way the child did. And that relationships don't have to follow the patterns that were laid down in her or his family.

Children also ask unanswerable questions. Magical though I am, I still can't answer things like "Why does God want this to happen to me?" So, I'm honest with the child about not knowing everything.

The longer the person stays with any experience, the more it collects its total components. Like the client who smelled cardboard. At first, he was only curious. I helped him to stay with that smell of cardboard. I asked him questions about it that could only be answered by staying with the experience. "Does it smell wet or dry?" I asked him questions like that. Some channel in his brain stayed open. And like a picture that comes slowly into focus or a tune you can't quite remember the words to, more and more of it came through until suddenly he was reliving a powerful experience. Every aspect of an experience is a route to the whole thing. To access the child state, I keep some channel open. As I ask for the components of a particular childhood experience, eventually an entire event begins to emerge. As part of that emergence, old feelings, gestures and ideas start coming back. The child who experienced all those things also comes back. The first hints of that child can appear before any clear memories of an event.

While I'm working with a client, thinking about who she is and how she got that way, I'm also tracking her in the here and now. I'm looking at facial expressions, postures, gestures. I'm listening to the tone of voice and sentence structure and I'm waiting for that child. Before I began waiting for and listening for the child, I'm sure I failed to notice its presence countless times. If you watch people in the subway, in restaurants, anywhere they are sitting quietly with nothing to do you can see the child there. Old friends when they meet are like little children. The child is very much part of us, closer to the surface than most people would imagine. "The child isn't something we outgrow, it is a lifelong channel for our spirit." Jon Eisman said that.

The child wants simple things. It wants to be listened to. It wants to be loved. It wants someone to play with. It doesn't want to have to do all kinds of dumb adult things before it's ready. It may not even know the words, but it wants its rights protected and its self-respect unviolated. So, what do we do when the child emerges? What kind of treatment does the child need? Well, the child doesn't need to beat on the bed. The child doesn't need to get into its pain and scream. It doesn't need to hyperventilate or say mantras and affirmations. The child needs something much simpler. It needs you to be there.

I want you to imagine what you would do if you had come upon that real child, in the original situation. What's a reasonable, compassionate thing to do for a child that's confused and upset? You sit and talk with the child. You listen. You find out what's bothering the child, you understand, comfort, hold the child in your arms; later, you play, you explain things, you tell a story. That's what the child needs, nothing fancy, just kindness and patience.

Usually, the child's confused. So you make a couple of contact statements, like, "I bet that really upsets you, huh?" You watch for the breath. The child starts to feel good as soon as it knows that you understand. Sometimes you have to talk about death. "You know, people die. It's nobody's fault. They get old and wear out." You might have to straighten out some of the child's ideas about people, love, sex, or whatever. You might help it to forgive someone. Anything you can do to get the child to feel better about itself. Any way you can help change a negative image the child may have gotten about itself. Just be a compassionate adult! Just take the time to talk to the child. It doesn't need any special techniques. The child will start to tell you what's bothering it as soon as it knows you care and are really listening. So, you're there and you're compassionate and the child starts to tell you what the problem is. It doesn't understand something. It feels bad about something. Sometimes, all you need to do is let the child tell you that. It just needed to tell somebody. Sometimes the child's perceptions need to be validated. The confusion is there because the adults tried to impose their view of things and it went against the child's true feelings about things. Sometimes, a child will just run up to you and say, "I fell down and I hurt my knee." "Yeah, I bet that really hurt, didn't it?" The child nods its head nine times and runs back to its playing. And that's enough. The child just wanted to tell somebody. Bursting with it, you know? Maybe it wanted to know if something should be done about it. "You know, I think it's okay. I think it will be all better in a little while."

The child state of consciousness dissolves as naturally as it appeared. When the work has been done, when the crying, listening, and thinking about it are done, maybe a little resting, too, then the work is over and ordinary consciousness returns. No fanfare. The signs of completion will be there and you'll be able to read them if you're looking for them. Just as this chapter ends.

12

GOING FOR MEANING

The expansion of consciousness does not lie in the quantitative accumulation of experiences, but in a qualitative change in the person experiencing.

Each time you climb to a higher vantage point the range of your vision is enlarged and your understanding of your entire situation is altered. You see things from a more encompassing perspective which allows you to be less concerned and anxious and enables you to relate to your environment in terms of how it really is rather than how you imagined it to be from a more limited point of view.

- Swami Rama and Swami Ajaya, Creative Use of Emotions

The goal of therapy is not any particular experience; it is a change which organizes all experiences differently, a change in the way of experiencing. To make that kind of change, we must deal with meanings and not just experiences. We must bring out the meaning of the way we organize experience, the way we do things, the way we put our world together, perceive it and think about it. We must search for meaning in the style of our interactions, the uses we make of our physical self, how and where we store tensions, which systems in the body take the stress. Posture, facial expressions, gestures, movement habits — all these have meanings. In short, all experiencing is embedded in and organized by images and beliefs, that is, by meanings.

Therapy doesn't stop when the client is in touch with his or her experience. It starts there. The therapist has to know both how to help the client get into and stay with experience and what to do with it. The most important thing to do with any important experience is to help the client to come to an understanding of it. The meaning of an experience is brought out in several ways: accessing memories associated with it; working with the feelings that link the experience to organizing beliefs; putting the experience into words, making the non-verbal, verbal. Describing the experience in words, transports it into the realms of symbol, imagination and thought where it can be studied, doubted, manipulated and reorganized.[1]

The techniques for going for meaning lead the client to specific, personal, individual, unique meanings and are part of a series of events that are that client's personal experience of therapy. The techniques are used to help the client understand how and why certain experiences are organized the way they are. For the therapist, understanding must be partly dictated by theory, such as that of character process. Therapy doesn't usually happen without something like that going on for the therapist. But, for the client, theory can easily be harmful. The therapist may need to understand the client partly in the general terms of some useful framework, just to move the therapy along, but the client needs to know himself or herself as fact — individual and personal. To offer general meaning to the client, to give the client labels to think about rather than experiences that enhance personal meaning, is to fail to appreciate the real nature of the therapeutic process. It's harder to come to specific meaning than to the general sort; it takes more time, intelligence and compassion. But for the well-being of the client, it's crucial.

An Example: The Technique of Going for Meaning Using Tension

Meaning is not just cognitive; it is embedded in experiences of all kinds. One kind is muscular tension. Tensions come up often in therapy, sometimes as responses to the evocation of experience, sometimes as the focus of the client's experienced difficulties. Sometimes people notice tensions as they slow down and become mindful. It comes up in everyone at sometime, but it is common for people who are sensory/motor encoders, people for whom their primary experiences are sensations and motor impulses. These people need and like to move and they habitually and unconsciously filter beliefs and emotions through their muscles. They may be experienced with studying their tensions for meaning. If they are, so much the better. If they're not, it's very easy to learn how tensions can be used to go for meaning.

Here is a general, four-step approach which can be used to go for meaning from tensions. Similar processes have been developed to go for meaning from other aspects of experience like feelings, memories, impulses, gestures, images, postures, movements, and sensations. Of course, you wait for the person to complete each step before going on the next. You may have to help some with the steps themselves through questions and contact statements.

1. Ask some deepening questions about the tension. Is the tension symmetrical? What kind of tension is it? What are its qualities? Questions like that. This stabilizes the experience and deepens contact with it. It is done in a quiet, relaxed state of mind, or in mindfulness. If necessary, repeat the probe or little experiment that evoked the tension in the first place.

2. Ask the person to notice any other parts of the body that participate or want to participate in the tension, like other tensions in the body, movements, words, sounds and so on. Again, repeat the probe or little experiment, if that works. This works to include the whole body. It is a step towards meaning because it takes the experience to a larger perspective. It takes it towards something the whole person is doing, not just a muscle or two.

3. The next step is to ask the person to do the tensing voluntarily, slowly, keeping mindfulness going by asking them to be careful to get it just right and do it a few times. Here is the step that takes the tension from involuntary to voluntary. This parallels the process of going from unconscious to conscious. It supports the transition to consciousness and therefore, to meaning.

4. Finally, when the pattern of tension in the whole body is clear and can be done voluntarily, ask the person to put words to what he or she is doing. "What are you saying with your body when you tense this way?" That sort of question. Emphasize that the words should come without effort or trying. The words should come spontaneously, or from the unconscious. And, they should fit. They should feel right to the person. When the words come up that way, they are often a clear expression of core material, especially if the original tension was part of a reaction to an important probe. They will be meaningful, which is what we were after in the first place.

To summarize this process: first deepen, then expand to the whole body, then make the tension(s) voluntary, then ask for meaning.

Meaning and Experience

Here are two specific examples of the possible meanings of tensions. One is tension in the eyes, the second, tension in the jaw. Tension in the eyes very often is a matter of not wanting to see something, like hatred in another's eyes, or to be seen or "seen into." It may also be searching for someone or for an answer to an important question. Or it could be blocked sadness. The meaning is personal; only the person who has the experience can declare its actual meaning. With the jaw, often it is anger or holding back expressing anger, not saying something. Or it could be resolve and determination. It might be keeping from being forced to accept something or to let something in.

Experiences in therapy are emotional and powerful. It takes time for the client to come through these to understanding. You'll need patience. You'll have to help the client come to his or her own discoveries. And even though you may have anticipated these discoveries, you'll have to use them "privately" to do the work of creating what's needed, so that the clients can come to them in their own way and time. You may feel the urge to take part more actively, to be visibly The Therapist. The truth is, it's much more effective to simply set the stage, to make the situation safe, to help access and support mindfulness and all the rest. That process will lead to discoveries, without taking from the client his or her achievement, that of self-discovery and change through determined and often painful effort. It takes courage to come to those discoveries and the client deserves to have and own them.

The whole point of therapy is change, change in the meaning we give to experience. So, we go for meaning in order to discover how we are creating it, what we are making out of what is given to us and to gain control of that process in order to give new meanings and create new experiences from them. We use experience to explore self-organization and to access core material. We use it to go from feelings and sensations and from muscles getting tense, to what those tensions are saying. The point is to access and change the symbolic world that shapes all experience. Of course the long-range goal of this pursuit of meaning is to recover the capacity to have full feelings and experiences without interrupting them, even to search for meaning. In the long run, the meaning and the experience are one and are sensed as such. It is only because some experiences are truncated, painful or confusing and somehow lack clear meaning that we have to go searching for it in the first place. It's because we value the freedom just to be that we do all this examining.

Meaning and Core Material

When the client is deeply involved, mindful and taking time with each step of the way, the process takes on a special quality. It is a living process, an unfolding. The therapist by then has probably developed some notions about what kind of process it is and what kind of probe or technique will work to bring the client into contact with core material. It's the therapist that has an idea about meanings and is experimenting with those meanings to access core material. A simple probe, at such times, can be all that's needed to bring on a deep, powerful experience for the client. The right words are like a key that suddenly opens the way to the client's very core.

An example: a client has been talking about burdens and restrictions and inescapable responsibilities. The therapist offers a probe like, "your life belongs to you." In reaction, the client feels and reports anger and disbelief and a tightening of the abdominals. So, you or your assistant take over that tightening and put some pressure on the abdominals to simulate the tension. Now you try the probe again, with the client letting you take over the tension in the abdominals, and now the reaction is an explosion of feeling and a clear memory, filled with rage and humiliation. The therapist asks, "what are you discovering or deciding in this memory?" With that question, the clear understanding comes that, "I cannot get the love I need if I feel and express this anger." With this insight, a recognition and a strong feeling of the truth of it come also. It makes sense of things.

We often attempt to access core material by going for the meaning of some bodily event. A bodily event that happens in reaction to a probe is, after all, part of a whole system of reactions, all organized and controlled by core beliefs, memories and so on. That intimate connection between reaction and core is what we use to access that material. The client realizes suddenly, that his body is saying, "touch me!" And with that, the feelings and the memories that make sense of that painful cry reveal themselves. In accessing core material this way, we go from present experience, sensations, feelings, thoughts, and so on, to beliefs, memories and images that, though they operate strongly and constantly on the present, are more a part of the hidden assumptions of the past.

There is more to do, of course, though just getting to meaning or core material can be a powerful event in a person's life. This is deep, formative material, at the center of who the client is and how he or she came to be that. To be in contact with and to understand these old events is to seem to arrive home, to know oneself in the most real and significant way. It is to feel and know the almost holy power to choose who one will be.

Notes for Chapter 12

1. Images themselves can be manipulated and reorganized in very fruitful ways. Healing can be done that way. When that happens, we can say that they have strong, unconscious meaning. They may not be translatable into words on the conscious level.

13

TRANSFORMATION, INTEGRATION AND COMPLETION

PART 1:

TRANSFORMATION

In fact, the laws governing conventional reality are flexible...

- Kalu Rinpoche, The Dharma

Of all the strange features of the universe, none are stranger than these: time is transcended, laws are mutable, and observer-participancy matters.

- John Wheeler

Learning is the discovery of the possible.

- Fritz Perls, The Gestalt Approach

At some point in processing, after emotions have been expressed, after the child has understood and gotten what she needs, after insight and meaning, a particular point is reached where the work of transformation takes place. A simple thing occurs. A seed is planted. The compelling grip of some piece of core material relaxes and new actions and experiences become possible. The discovery of that possibility is the transformation. What is new is that one can be different; one's whole life can be different. The point of transformation in therapy is the point where the client knows this and takes actions based upon this knowledge, and finds that these actions work.

It may be that the transformation begins with the client accepting a new belief, a belief like: I'm okay the way I am. Or it may be that the transformation begins with expressing something, like anger or love, something the client has a habit of holding back. Then, in the safe, comfortable setting of therapy, the client experiments with her new options. The client studies her options, noticing their effects. The experiences around transformation can be a great relief and a delicious pleasure. After all, the client has been waiting for years to do or say or feel or believe this thing. It's new only in the sense that it is an option that hasn't been taken up till now. All along, it's been waiting, embedded in its opposite.

The Experience That Wants to Happen

In any authoritarian model of healing, the client is a problem to be solved. In Hakomi, the client is an experience that wants to happen. It should have happened in the normal course of growth, but it didn't. The goal of therapy is to coax that experience into happening. What follows is a list of the missing core experiences for each character process. See Chapter 3, the section entitled The Experience That Wants to Happen.

Like Perls' "aha" or Feldenkrais' spontaneous reorganization, the transformation is often spontaneous. It feels and looks like transformation. I worked with a woman once, in a workshop. She did some things about birth and safety and just being here. It had a lot to do with not having to hide, and that meant opening her eyes and just looking around without searching for what was going to get her. We worked in the morning. All the rest of that day, I'd see her wide-eyed with wonder, looking at things, trees out the window, flowers in a vase, people's faces. She was living her new eyes. Once you've lived a new, powerful and beautiful experience like that, you are transformed. You know the old and the new and you want the new. Why keep going to a closed restaurant having found one that's open?

As the client tries out and savors the new belief or behavior, the face is visibly changed. It is open and often childlike, or at least it is younger. It is relaxed or flushed with energy. Smiles aren't unknown. I worked one weekend at the Primal Therapy Institute of Denver. During some work with a man stuck in a deep sensitive-analytic process, we came slowly, over the course of an hour and a half, to a place where the terror of expressing himself gave way to the joy of it. He was jumping into the air. We held onto him and helped him jump, up into the air. And he was making sweet sounds of joy with every leap. The sounds weren't loud and they weren't forced in any way. They were just escaping from him like steam from a pot of happy soup. A woman next to me, a therapist at that institute for seven years, turned to me and said, "We've never heard that sound in this building before."

In Hakomi, we pursue transformation. That is the goal of therapy: to learn and master new options. It is by savoring them and adding to them that the client comes to know and value them above his previous behaviors. Thus, the client comes to incorporate and integrate new beliefs and ways of being. As the change completes, the client may experience a flow of insights and memories or go in and out of the rapids. Each must be given its time. It's a bit like tidying up after the big game. Transformation is a process.

PART 2:

INTEGRATION

T he work in therapy is just the seed of transformation. The new beliefs, feelings, and perceptions have to be taken out into the world. To survive, the transformation must find support. In therapy, we do our best to give it a good start. We spend some time integrating.

Integration involves getting used to, making connections and finding a place for the new thing in the larger scheme of things. So, we spend some time trying new behaviors out and noticing the effects. For example, we might try a probe that was an important part of the process to see how it was reacted to now. If it is taken in as nourishing and feels good, we can repeat a few times to allow more and more aspects of the experience to become clear. That helps integrate the new belief. In a workshop, I might have other people offer the nourishing statement for the same reason. That is a passive way of integrating and it's often done in mindfulness. Active expression is also done, but less so since we are interested in core beliefs changing and they are more clearly reflected by automatic reactions. Actions are voluntary and deliberate. Therefore, they can be very misleading about core material that way.

Some integration occurs unconsciously. If the session has been a powerful one, as many are, it's a good idea to give the client space and time right then to rest quietly, talking, if she likes, starting to understanding more and more of the

implications of the discoveries made. This restful period immediately after a
session has a strong, integrating influence. Sleep, when that feels right, has the
same quality. The long-term aspects of integration take place over weeks, months
and years. Once a change has started, it needs to be stabilized. It needs to be
integrated into the client's life. Since the feelings, thoughts and actions are new
and very different from what the client has been used to, the client's relationships,
with family members, friends and work associates will all be under some strain.
The client isn't just changing herself. She is changing how she relates to
everyone. The world doesn't let you change that much, so easily. What the
change itself has going for it is that it feels good and has been made conscious.
In the microcosm of the therapy session, the client now needs support for the
changes he is making. The therapist is the first person available for that.

In the following paragraphs, I describe several ways to support and integrate
the transformation.

Savoring. Within a therapy session, when a client first accepts a nourishing
belief and is first trying it out, I encourage the client to savor the experience,
especially the good feelings that arise out of it. As with accessing, it's a matter
of staying with the new experience and giving it time to become clear, to make
connections to it. I try to keep the client focused on the experience. I ask questions
about it or if the child is there, I play games with it. I sometimes suggest to the
client that she simply let the unconscious yield up images and memories that make
sense of the experience. Here are several more ways to help the client to savor
the changes that follow transformation:

(1) Ask the client to compare the nourishment offered in words with what
happens when touch is used. There is often a strong difference in accepting and
believing between verbal and physical expressions of the same thing, especially
if people in the past weren't honest with the child. (2) If you're working in a group,
you can let the client hear the nourishing statement from many voices, one at a
time. If you are alone with the client, you can have her imagine significant people
in her life offering that nourishment. Always, the experience is studied. (3) You
can ask the client to look for ways to make the nourishment even better or more
satisfying. The usual result of asking for refinement or precision is a deepening
of concentration and an enhancement and stabilizing of the experience. (4) If
you've been working with the child, you can ask the client to imagine holding the
child and giving it nourishment.

Using Mindfulness. The habits around taking in and keeping out nourishment
can also be studied mindfully. The client can do that first by noticing what he or
she does involuntarily with the nourishing statement or touch. Then the client can

experiment with controlling the reaction deliberately, first closing down against the nourishment, shutting it out, then taking it in and savoring it. The effects of both become much clearer and the preference for one over the other is strongly established. Using mindfulness, the client can imagine all sorts of situations that can and probably will come up, such as having to maintain the new attitudes and feelings with relatives and friends, at home and at work. Taking one person at a time and imagining being with that person while feeling nourished in the particular way just discovered can help reveal what will be needed from each person to help integrate these new things.

One can also compare present feelings to those which arose before in situations evocative of the old beliefs. Studying almost any aspect of the process of integration, especially with mindfulness, will help to integrate it, particularly in the early stages of that process.

Appreciating the Child. People are often angry at themselves for living under a negative belief. They need to understand that, in the child's world, those old beliefs were a necessary framework from which to operate. They need to appreciate and understand not only the pain and suffering of the child, but also the creativity and resourcefulness the child showed. We can do this by simply talking about it, or showing our own appreciation for the child or by telling a story in the fashion of Milton Erickson, a story which demonstrates, without saying so directly, how creative and adaptive children are and need to be.

Bringing It All Back Home. Some of the things we do in the office are directed at clarifying the work that has be done in the world outside the office. Some ways to deal with that are: (1) Provide time after the therapy session to be alone in order to absorb the experience, to rest and think about it. You can advise clients not to schedule any work activity after a therapy session. A hot tub and a massage are even better. (2) In fantasy, the client can relive his or her whole life assuming the new belief and support for it from everyone around. (3) The client can examine the past for times when such nourishment was given or offered, emphasizing that it is available in the outside world. The client may practice asking for just what he or she wants, by role playing a situation where the old belief might interfere. (4) The client can also consciously experiment with the postural changes involved in going from old belief to new. (5) You talk about taking it home, what that's going to be like, how others may react, and how it all came to be. This bit of discussion and analysis will help the client find some things to think about and to talk about with some of the people she is close to. These are just a few ways taking it home can be supported. There are many others waiting to be discovered, invented and tried.

Housekeeping. During any session, times arise when the therapist needs to give and get some feedback on how the session itself is going. Though important for several reasons, housekeeping can also be integrating. It can help clarify the events of the session. It also provides an opportunity for the client to spend some time away from the intense concentration of the main process. Since most of the main process takes place in states other than ordinary consciousness, the recapitulation of events in those states helps to integrate them. This interruption of the ongoing process at appropriate points is not disruptive, it is a necessary rest which offers time and space to go over what one has done and to learn from it. The most appropriate times to do this type of housekeeping are when the client seems to come naturally to a place of rest.

As long as we're talking about housekeeping, let's talk about what else it is good for. It is useful when the therapist feels unclear about what's really happening or feels some tension or strain between herself and the client. If I feel I'm not getting the cooperation of the unconscious or that the client doesn't view our roles in therapy the same way I do, I will house keep that. Often, some point about the process itself would be helpful to the client, perhaps to explain the nature of a special kind of intervention or one the client is likely to be unfamiliar with. Housekeeping is much like jumping out of the system (chapter 19) and is one of the ways to do that. It refocuses the session on those things that are keeping the session from going along smoothly. The process recovers quite easily and naturally from such housekeeping interruptions and profits from them in the long run.

Homework. I give people things they can do outside the office or after the workshop. These tasks can help to stabilize new behaviors and are especially powerful around relationships, images of self and behaviors no longer wanted. Homework can include changes in diet or bodywork (like massage, Rolfing, exercise, movement, yoga, Feldenkrais work); keeping a journal; or something special for a particular situation. For example, I once asked a woman using a burdened-enduring strategy, a strategy fueled by guilt, to stand all day in Kenmore Square in Boston (the main subway interchange) wearing a sign that read, "IT'S ALL MY FAULT." I heard she did it and I heard she had a great time, talking to people, getting questions and advice and a lot of laughs. I can easily imagine how it could have changed her.

PART 3:

COMPLETION

Sometimes sessions seem to go on and on, never coming to a natural ending. It doesn't happen often, but when it does it's a problem. Most sessions have a way of coming to an appropriate closing easily and spontaneously. But once in a while, ending the session will be difficult, especially with certain character processes, like clinging-expressive or dependent-endearing. It usually happens when the session has dealt with more superficial stuff and the deeper issue of separation wasn't handled. Some people want don't want the therapy session to end, it feels like separation or loss to them. Some of the ways to handle situation are as follows: (1) House keep it. Point it out and discuss it. Offer your thoughts about what's happening. If they don't feel complete, perhaps they can accept that and make it something to work on next time. (2) If the completion problem is part of an expressive-clinging process and you don't want to keep working or get into a long discussion about things, it's often best to just begin the closure process yourself. You can do that by making a statement that implies that the session will be ending soon. Like, "I'll tell you a story before we stop." Or you can ask a question like, "what would you like to do before we stop?"

Usually, a good session comes to a close naturally. The intensity subsides and changes from working and being highly focused to just sitting around and talking in a normal conversational tone of voice over a wider range of topics. That's a good sign that the session completed organically. That's the best. Because therapy can be so intense, some people have a little trouble coming back to the everyday world. Just talking, maybe over a cup of tea, or taking a walk for a half hour will help.

SECTION THREE

THE METHOD

Nothing else matters half so much.
To reassure one another,
To answer each other.

Everyone has, inside himself
- what shall I call it?
A piece of good news!

Ugo Betti

14

BASIC JOBS

PART 1:

BASIC JOBS

There are a few basic jobs that govern this therapy process. Therapists need to understand and master them. They comprise two major tasks, managing the ongoing process and gathering information. These two jobs are interdependent. They can enhance one another or, as happens all too frequently, they interfere with each other. These are two broad, important responsibilities. We need to manage what's going on. We need to do something to keep the process on track. Actually, many things. For example, we need to know when to take charge and how much and just as often, when to lay off and let things move along without interference. We need to know how to recognize when things aren't going well and how to recover from that. That's all part of managing the process. There is also a great deal to learn about gathering information.

Managing the Process

This is the primary job, all else depends upon it. We must let gathering information be secondary. We must let curiosity wait for answers or find our answers silently, by observing. Our primary responsibility is to support the unfolding process of the client. If we have questions we want answered, they must be secondary to this unfolding. All too often, we ask questions when we should be making contact or just remaining silent. This interferes with what the other needs or wants to do. When we indulge ourselves with too many questions, the situation quickly becomes one in which the client feels they are there to be "worked on," to wait for questions, to answer them and to wait again either for another question or to be told what to do next. That won't work to unlock experiences that need to happen. This setup does as much to block the unfolding process as anything else I've ever seen, including the repressions of the unconscious.

Managing the process involves interventions of all types and a sense of when to use which. It can be either passive and active. It requires a subtle balance between taking charge and directing the process and stepping back and leaving room for the other to choose the direction taken. This stepping back involves being silent at critical times, waiting and allowing the other to lead. Active management requires interventions like contact, accessing, deepening, jumping out of the system and housekeeping. Passive management requires stepping back and allowing client time to tell his or her story or just to think or integrate. The other should have a sense of spaciousness, a sense that he or she has lots of time and has the primary influence on how the process of therapy unfolds. For this the therapist must be tracking for when the other is consciously or unconsciously choosing a direction and at those times must simply be silent.

Managing the process also involves managing states of consciousness. That means tracking for them, evoking new ones, and moving from one state of consciousness to another. In a typical session, the client will start in ordinary consciousness and will need at some point to move into mindfulness or into the child or emotional processing. That's what usually happens. The therapist has to follow and detect when it is time to move from one state to the other. It's a matter of getting the feel for it, getting a sense of when one phase is complete and another is ready and knowing how to support those changes with interventions.

Once the client has told her story, the next thing can happen. At that point, it's a good idea to take charge and have something to try - a probe, for example. First, acknowledge the story by making some summary contact statement about it. Then it's good to ask if it is now a good time to try some exploring or deepening. If the other person feels like it might be, the next thing to do is to ask for mindfulness and support it with change in pace and tone of voice. Then do the little experiment or whatever. That's when, and a little about how, to go from ordinary consciousness to mindfulness. The movement into processing states is similar. You work from signs that the time is ripe. Either you hear and see the child or feelings emerging. The time to go for meaning is when the client becomes curious after touching the child state or the emotional state.

Other important management jobs involve deciding what to do when the process derails or looks like it's going to derail. I call this "staying in the game." Again, it requires a feel for what's happening and what's needed.

It requires knowing when:

> the client still has more to tell
> the client is done telling her story
> to introduce mindfulness
> to access, to deepen, to experiment
> to stop experimenting
> to simply offer nourishment
> you're not going slow enough
> the client needs to slow down
> safety needs are up
> to be silent

and knowing how to:

> turn the client inward
> support the shift to mindfulness
> let the client know you're on his/her side
> get the client to report present experience
> get the client to stay with present experience

and getting a feel for when the client:

> can't stay with experience
> reacts rather than responds
> avoids responsibility
> is only into feeling and:
> has no interest in the meaning
> is only into meaning and:
> has little feeling about any of it
> doesn't reveal important present experiences
> has strong reactions to being led
> is unable to understand mindfulness
> has little or no distance on their own experience

and noticing problems, like:

> frequent interruptions of the process
> delays in the flow of the process
> hostility towards the therapist
> low energy levels
> unstoppable verbal production

Much of this, like pace and strategies, needs to be adjusted to the individual client. They're all unique.

In any nonviolent psychotherapy, directing, leading and in general, taking charge is going to be a sensitive and subtle process. Violence and taking charge are not the same thing. Nonviolence is about how you act, not whether you act. It isn't violent simply to take action or to direct. In fact, sometimes it is more violent not to take action. It is only violent to force action against the wishes or resistance of the other. It is violent to take sides when taking sides is divisive and destructive. If you can act in a way that's consistent with the client's felt needs and your own, if you track carefully, understand the best you can, use appropriate timing and get permission on all levels from both the client and yourself, your actions will be nonviolent.

Within those limits, you can take charge. If you constantly track for how your suggestions and directions are being received, you can always back off as soon as something feels like it is against the grain. Then you are being nonviolent. Taking charge is then as simple as offering suggestions or giving direct commands. For example, "stay with that sadness for a while and notice what it wants." Taking charge may also mean asking the person to stay with something painful. That means you must be willing to see them in their pain. Pain is full of information about what's wrong and what's needed. Staying with pain is sometimes the best way to learn from it. The client's habits are most likely to be ways to avoid or escape the pain, so staying with it may help us learn something. If you try to alleviate the pain too quickly, you'll most likely fail to contact and understand the core material behind the pain and nothing much will change.

Lastly, it wise to remember these things: (1) you are only in charge of the process of therapy, which is secondary (at least for the client) to the processes of staying alive and being who they are and taking care of, protecting and enhancing themselves; (2) you cannot heal the other, only support their own healing process. So, don't insist on your agendas; if you violate the client's priorities, like safety and control, the process will derail. You must be willing to back off.

Some Obvious Signs That Something Else Is Needed

STAGES   SIGNS

1. relationship building

   trust/safety   client is guarded, nervous, can't go
                          inside, body contracted, arms folded
                          across body, head turned slightly to side

   unconscious   client answers too quickly, or
                          doesn't give serious, considered
                          answers, goes blank, misinterprets,

2. therapy mode

   mindfulness   client is reactive, abstracting,
   internal focus   externally focused, into problem
                          solving, high levels of verbal
                          production and speed, needs to talk
                          all the time, is too focused on
                          therapist as "savior", expert, to
                          go inside,

   slowing down   client doesn't stay with an
                          experience, new interests emerge
                          when you try to deepen, client goes
                          blank, comes out of mindfulness

Gathering Information

Gathering information is secondary to managing the process. It must be done primarily by tracking and thinking. As I've mentioned before, we must be careful to avoid leading the client this way and that in order to satisfy our curiosity. That sort of thing can easily derail therapy by taking the client out of his or her own process. So, the therapist gathers information while avoiding too much direct help from the client. This information gathering uses few questions and suggests in its general demeanor that the time belongs to the other, for his or her purposes.

So, we learn about the client by tracking present experience, by listening for beliefs, by sensing the systematic and tracking the therapist-client relationship. We do it by creating and doing little experiments, thereby evoking all kinds of experiences which therapist and client study.

A therapist is his or her own instrument, just as a musician or an actor or an athlete is. So, we use our own experience, allowing our feel of the relationship to come clearly into verbal consciousness. This makes it possible to jump out of the system. Sometimes we "try on" the client's experience, by momentarily taking on the client's posture, gestures feelings and/or facial expressions, to feel what it's like to be in the client's world right now. This trying on gets to be second nature and involves little or no actual movement. These are high skills; they need to be mastered. They are essential. Eudora Welty said, "it's much harder to listen *for* a story than *to* a story." Therapists do hard things like that.

We also have a strong influence on the way the client gathers information. We do it by modeling mindfulness, precision, slow pace, curiosity, being in the present, searching for the meaning in tensions; by all the ways we express the principles. This modeling is a primary influence on the client. We do it by:

> using contact statements rather than questions
> sometimes, simply listening, without needing to direct
> teaching mindfulness
> teaching about the search for meaning and core beliefs
> directing the process towards present experience
> directing the process towards the organization of experience
> keeping the channels open
> deepening, rather than jumping around
> not jumping into explanations and theories
> going for meaning
> keeping an experimental, information gathering attitude.

There are some important things to wonder about during the ongoing process, things like: what role is the client choosing for him or herself? What role are you being put in? Where is the process going? What wants to happen? What kind of system are we getting into? Just wondering and being curious, without actively pursuing information will build the attitudes and habits that make for strong intuitions. Also, staying with and following the client's interests and curiosity will teach you about the underlying orderliness on which both you and the client can rely. That in turn builds faith in the effortless emergence of what is needed for our healing and growing, and all the experiences that are waiting to happen.

What We Focus On

The method works with both experience and beliefs. Beliefs, especially emotionally charged beliefs, direct, organize, and limit experiences. So each present experience is an immediate example of the organizing power of beliefs. We work with experience in order to reach core beliefs, to bring them into consciousness where we can explore alternatives. We work with alternative beliefs in order to create the possibility of new experiences. We go back and forth between experience and belief. We sometimes call that working at the mind-body interface. By staying with a particular experience long enough, memories, beliefs and meaningful images arise. By staying with images, memories and beliefs in an open way, experiences rich in feeling arise. The movement in therapy is back and forth between these two levels.

The method uses nourishment in several ways. One way is touch. We touch and hold clients, when they're in pain, sad, expressing the hurt child. We also offer nourishing statements. One use is to explore, in mindfulness, how the other organizes around the opportunity of nourishment. After all, if you are not getting what you need from life, there are only two possibilities: either the world doesn't have it (in which case, therapy won't help you get it) or the world does have it and you aren't taking it. We like to discover and work with the nourishment that's available and isn't being taken in. We explore the beliefs that prevent the taking in.

We also use nourishment to build strength and courage. By offering such things as kind words, touching and holding, we help clients get ready for the often difficult emotional work that therapy can be. And, in all this we are careful not to give nourishment that is not taken in. That is our safeguard against creating dependencies. We are tracking, when we offer nourishment, whether the other really takes it in or not. Sometimes, the other is more attracted to the idea of nourishment and the role playing around that than in the actual, physical experiences of pleasure, relief, warmth, etc. In those cases, we use mindfulness to focus on the issue of nourishment. If the nourishment is being taken in, the experience will include satisfaction and completion. Real nourishment always completes. It is accepted and assimilated. Sooner or later, it fulfils the need it supplies and a reorientation takes place. Many good sessions end with a period of time where the client takes in some type of nourishment he or she could not take in before. And for a while, it seems like they can not get enough of it. But, after ten or fifteen minutes usually, the client becomes interested in completing and moving on to something else. The process comes to a spontaneous and ordinary end. If we are careful with nourishment and use mindfulness when clarity is needed, dependency becomes something to study or is avoided completely.

We also work a great deal with the body. As I mentioned just above, we work at the mind-body interface. We go back and forth between bodily experiences and the meaning of those experiences. For example, we will use a probe and then study the experience it evokes, like tension somewhere, or sensations. Alternatively, we may take a bodily experience, like tension, and go for the meaning by asking the person to allow the unconscious to provide words, images or memories that are related to the tension. Of course, it all has to be done with the appropriate timing and phrasing. The connection to the unconscious has to be there. We also track for bodily signs of inner experience through gesture, posture, facial expression and even body structure, color, texture, temperature and movement style. All these are a constant reference for whatever effects our interventions are having.

In addition to these, as described in previous chapters, we work with specific states of consciousness and the organization of experience.

PART 2:

THE LOGIC OF THE METHOD

*I*ntroduction. The method we use is to find a route to core material in order to modify its influence on the client's life. We attempt to find, through the client's present experience - posture, body structure, gesture, tone of voice - clues to the client's core material and routes to access that material. I think of this as working with information processes, in living systems. Such a perspective helps generate the method's logic. It helps us describe and clarify the assumptions upon which the work is based. It's from these assumptions that our way of working with people has developed.

Hakomi is a clearly defined and teachable way of working with people. Though much art goes into using the method, much sensitivity and creativity, the underlying logic is pragmatic and explicit. We have in Hakomi, a full curriculum of theory and several hundreds of hours of experiential exercises. I and the other trainers and teachers have taught people to do Hakomi for over ten years now.

The method concerns itself with the way people process information. There are two sets of information involved. One maintains and enhances biological organization. The other maintains symbolic organization, including language, self image and cultural influences. The interaction of these two systems, mind and body, creates and maintains the whole set of operations we call character. Therefore we focus on and use particularly information at the mind-body interface, information that integrates and flows between the symbolic and biological processes. The method is therefore body-centered, and one of its main goals is to create a harmonious interaction between these two basic systems.

The view of healing taken is one in which the therapist follows and supports the organic processes of the other, processes in which the need for self-regulation is essential. The client is not just an information processing system. The client, in the most technical and scientific sense, is a living system. So, the method is not just body-centered, it is living-centered. And because we humans are very special living systems in this part of the solar system, having uniquely important symbolic and cultural capacities, the method is self-consciously human centered. Like Taoists of old we abhor going against the grain, using force when it simply isn't needed. Ours is a beautifully energy efficient, nonviolent, nontoxic "medicine."

Our goals are to encourage, support and create change at the level of core material. In approaching this goal we do not struggle with the defenses. We actually support them. We view them as efforts to manage experience. In supporting them we are working to create a relationship in which the other will feel safe enough to yield voluntarily to the experience and expression of core memories and emotions. All of us avoid contact with core material by creating noise in the form of distractions and diversions, by focusing elsewhere and keeping our levels of tension high enough to mask feelings and reduce sensitivity. Safety lowers the noise and the focus on present experience brings us into contact with the core.

Assumptions

The method is grounded in these assumptions about information processes and people: Any experience contains access routes to the biological and symbolic structures that support it. These routes begin with aspects of the experience itself, like sensations, feelings, thoughts, images, impulses, etc. Support structures help create and organize experience while remaining for the most part outside of awareness.

Staying with a particular experience, gathering more information by keeping the experience alive and exploring more and more of the immediate, present, mostly bodily aspects, will eventually and automatically contact and access its support structures. One can increase the amount of information about a particular, active experience in two ways. The first way is to spend more time in the experience. Information accumulates over time. More time, more information. The other way is this: increase sensitivity. We can increase the amount of information we get from any experience by bringing sensitivity to a high level and keeping it there. In Hakomi, we increase and maintain sensitivity primarily through techniques which lower noise rather than raise signal levels. Since all character processes involve habits which keep the client from becoming too sensitive to his or her own inner process, we find ways to:

Come in under the radar. Support structure information is normally unconscious, allowing full consciousness to attend to the experience being supported. For example, heart rate and breathing and the rules of sentence structure all influence speech, but they do so outside awareness and for the most part go unnoticed. The processes that keep core material from consciousness are similar. Rather than using aggressive techniques which arouse these consciousness management processes, we support the whole person, especially safety needs, thereby entering into the client's processes as an ally. We lower the noise, thereby increasing sensitivity. We stay with experience. We use gentleness and time.

THE LIFE CENTRAL FUNCTIONS

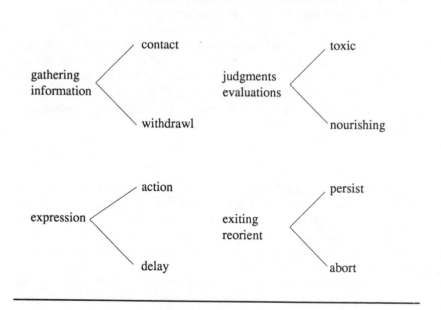

Gathering information is intimately connected to the functions around distancing, orienting and inclusion. Expression is similarly tied to control and impulsivity, judgment to affection, attachment and appreciation. The three variables - inclusion, control and affection - are the ones used by William Schutz in his analysis of personality and anxiety (2). We associate the exit function with creating and maintaining organized and integrated hierarchies of needs and wants. It is about giving each task its due, neither more nor less, and balancing rest with activity.

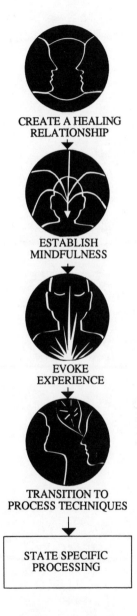

Compare with page 72.

THE SENSITIVITY CYCLE

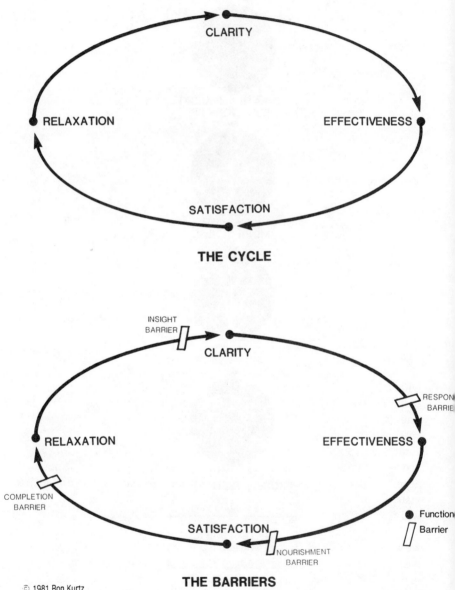

CLARITY

RELAXATION

EFFECTIVENESS

SATISFACTION

THE CYCLE

INSIGHT
BARRIER

CLARITY

RESPON
BARRIE

RELAXATION

EFFECTIVENESS

COMPLETION
BARRIER

SATISFACTION

● Function

▱ Barrier

NOURISHMENT
BARRIER

THE BARRIERS

15

LOWERING THE NOISE:
THE SENSITIVITY CYCLE

I n psychophysics there's a law called the Weber-Fechner Law. It states that the level of signal you can detect is dependent on the background noise. The more background noise, the more signal you will need. This simple, obvious law tells us something about helping people get in touch with themselves. We don't have to analyze their problems and tell them what's going on. We don't have to force any experiences on them. We don't have to make them feel. We can simply help them get the noise down. As the noise goes down, the signal emerges.

As you can no doubt tell, I embrace the notion that healing is directed from within, that it is organic. This is true on all levels, especially the psychological. In therapy, we want to turn the client inward, to help the client go deep inside, to find direction and meaning from somewhere deep within, from the core. To change at the level of the core is difficult. We have habits which avoid bringing core material, especially traumatic material, into consciousness. We learned long ago to redirect awareness if we even get close to such things. If we attempt to go deeply into ourselves, focusing on some experience organized by painful core material, we will have difficulties tuning in to it. Distractions, tensions, anxieties will flood our awareness, interrupting our search.

We can make an analogy here. The material we wish to focus on is a signal we wish to tune in.. The distractions, tensions, and anxieties which interfere are noise that blocks the signal. A system with a lot of noise will need a strong signal in order for anything to be perceived. Like a candle in the sun, or a whisper at a rock concert, a low level of signal won't be seen or heard. If we want to change that, there are only two things we can do: we can raise the signal or lower the noise. We can raise the signal by making a bonfire instead of using a candle, or by yelling, rather than whispering. In therapy, that usually means increasing the level of intensity, for example, by exaggerating expressions of feeling. The second way to change the situation is to lower the noise, to wait until dark to light your candle or to have the rock musicians and audience quiet down. You probably can't do that at a real concert, but you can if you're listening on your stereo. In therapy, lowering the noise means handling safety issues, relaxing, taking the effort out, taking over, becoming mindful. In Hakomi, we have a strong preference for lowering the noise, rather than raising the signal. As you lower the noise in any system, it becomes more sensitive, it is able to hear or see or feel or remember better.

The sensitivity cycle is a model for how we lower the noise in Hakomi, how we help clients to get to the information that's within. It uses many techniques which help the client cycle through a series of stages in order to become more and more sensitive. As the client becomes increasingly sensitive, either the information within becomes clearer or the habits which manage experience take over and interrupt the cycle of increasing sensitivity. In which case, they become clearer. We are then better able to understand and handle these blocks, to give them the time and attention they need, and get them back to the cycle. When we reach the core this way, through increasing sensitivity, we open to the possibility of choice at that deepest level. Choice at the level of the core is very special.

We are self-creating, self-maintaining, self-organized beings. Our development unfolds from within. It has an identity; it knows what is self and what is not. It can repair itself. It can heal. All living systems are organized this way, from single cell beings on up. We have created and are maintaining who we are as expressions of our kind. The core is this level of identity and self-organization, at least in the psychological sense, perhaps beyond. So it is important to know how we do that — how we self-organize and maintain and how we heal when we've been damaged.

This self that we self-created started with several things, our genetic inheritance, our "initial organizing configuration," to use David L. Shapiro's term for the original emotional and physical environment. We unfold from a certain starting place, from temperament and inherited potential. We start in simple ways, growing more and more complex, building each new level on what we achieved in organization and integration at the level below. Childhood introduced the themes which are now the attitudes, beliefs, opinions, strategies and habits of the present person. Just as the first step of a journey is more significant for the direction it announces than the distance it covers, our early patterns are important because they set the course that has shaped everything which followed and finally became the form and style of the self we are today.

First we learn a self and then, for the rest of our lives, we simply use it. As children, we make a map of who we are and who we love and how we will communicate. We make a map of what kind of world it is, what's possible in it and what isn't. Then as adults we go around using our map without changing it much. At first we are map makers, then map users. In this analogy, I am using Julian Jaynes' images and ideas from his book, *The Origins of Consciousness in the Breakdown of the Bicameral Mind*. But the map maker and the map user are doing very different things. In childhood, we make the self; as adults, we use it. As adults, we maintain through habit the self we created long ago. Those acts of self-creation are forgotten. When we are using the self, we do not feel it as changeable. The more our world threatens to change the self, the more energy we use to stabilize it. But it is changeable. All of our strongly held beliefs were once new ideas and doubtable. All our tired old habits were once just things we were trying out, playing with, even those that seem unbreakable now. The self was once fresh and flexible. Within us there is still that possibility of re-creation. Deep within, the maker of the self remains. The child map-maker is still a part of us. His blueprints are there. They can all be reexamined. It is by increasing sensitivity that we reach the map, the map maker and the possibility of change. By accessing the core, we find not just the created self but the power that creates.

This turning inward to study the self takes special conditions and guidance. It requires time and care and support. To make the search within, we need mindfulness and a calm, unhurried attitude. Effort, struggle, goals and a focus on achievements make mindful attention difficult. (Think of monasteries.) Self-discovery requires a meditative attitude. You cannot storm the self. Force will not work. Force sends the map maker into hiding. Battles are fought by map users. There is no time for wonder and creation when the gates are under siege, when the self needs defending. No! For studying the self, for going within, for leaving walls and battlements behind, peace is needed. Gentleness, time and support are needed. Nonviolence, love, the presence of supportive people, another kind of courage - these blessings are needed. Only they yield up the self so that it may be known and changed. And nothing else does it.

As living beings we have a natural aptitude for organizing ourselves efficiently. Efficiency has survival value and it feels good. It seems only natural for an organism to monitor its behavior for effectiveness and economy, dropping the extraneous, useless, and wasteful components of its actions. It's the same for us. When we're mindful, monitoring our actions, watching the how of our movements, perceptions, and reactions, we automatically get better at what we're doing. Mastery is the natural result of mindfulness. The work of Moshe Feldenkrais is based on this tendency we have of ordering ourselves in the most effective way, given the chance. In teaching people to function better, Feldenkrais repeats a pattern of movement, over and over again, in quiet, effortless ways, sometimes asking questions that keep the person in his or her experience. In that repetition, in that staying with a particular experience, discovering what is happening, we become aware of and sensitive to the details of our actions. Out of this awareness, we build new and easier ways to move, and a new body-image, more pleasure, more aliveness. And with this comes a new image of the self. Feldenkrais called his work *Awareness Through Movement* and wrote a book by that name. Through becoming aware of, repeating and differentiating a movement pattern, we become more aware of the many different ways we could do things and quite naturally, we automatically select the more effective, efficient and pleasurable ways. These two things — effective action and awareness — complement each other. Awareness helps you become effective and effectiveness, which makes things generally easier, allows you more time and energy to use your awareness. It can become a cycle, each part feeding the next, increasing effectiveness and awareness over and over again. In a slightly more elaborate form, this is the sensitivity cycle.

Here's the basic cycle. Awareness, mindfulness, attention, insight, (gathering information), makes action more effective. It makes for more effective responses to the situation. Of course it does. Think of walking around with your eyes closed. When we respond more effectively, we get more positive results like more nourishment, satisfaction, and pleasure. Satisfaction eventually allows for the completion of our actions around whatever need we were responding to. That is, as a need is satisfied, we relax our efforts. This relaxation, in turn, increases the potential for awareness. Relaxation is a dropping of effort and that, as we shall see soon, means less noise. Less noise, more sensitivity. Less noise, more awareness. That's the complete cycle, from awareness to effective responses to nourishment, to completion and the dropping of effort, to a new, higher level of awareness.

Wonder, experiment, openness, these promote change. Habit, the trance of ordinary consciousness, the intense pursuit of narrow goals, these destroy our natural potential for healthy reorganization. Narrow attention and rapid action are quite necessary, at times, when it is important that we reach some goal without disruption. Think of a rushing to the hospital with a woman in labor. No time there for quietly studying one's subtle reactions. Just keep your mind on the job and get safely through the traffic. Yes! For that kind of thing, speed and focused attention are just the ticket. For studying the self, it won't work. For studying the self, the time needs eyes that need not watch the road.

Sensitivity and Emotional Material

Somewhere I have a slide of an enormously fat man walking alone on a quiet, late afternoon street, past a small, delicate, blossoming tree. I used to go out and stalk the wild character types with my camera. This fat man was one of my prize catches. He must weigh four hundred pounds. He's round, from his knees to his ears. He's built like a squash standing on its thinner end. There is something very beautiful about him - he's perfectly balanced. He appears to be floating down the street. That four-hundred pound body looks as light and graceful and moves as effortlessly as any ballerina. He seems shy and is moving quickly, as if he didn't want to be seen. He and the tree are contrasts in grace. I am amazed each time I see him frozen in that beautiful moment. It's the delicacy, the lightness of him, the way he seems to float. He is exquisitely balanced. And, when you think about it, he has to be. It's the only way he could carry that much weight. If he leaned even a little bit too much in any direction, he would fall over.

His need for balance taught me something about experiencing. To experience deeply, you have to be balanced. If you're out of balance, with any sensitivity, strong experiences overwhelm you. In therapy, as sensitivity increases, whatever imbalances we have tip our processes into diversion or emotional chaos. From dealing honestly and courageously with that chaos, we learn to recover our balance. We improve our abilities to stay clear and upright and graceful, under even the gross burden of what in the long run is simply, the human condition.

My ideas about getting to the deeper beliefs in people are very simple. As one relaxes, with awareness gently focused on present experience, sensitivity increases and attempts to manage the experience slowly yield to the acceptance of whatever emerges. At some point in this process, we reach a level of sensitivity where experience becomes intense and emotional. Until one is clear and balanced, this emergence of emotional material will have to happen. The only way to avoid it is to either stay tense, and therefore insensitive, or to look somewhere else, to shift your awareness to something else. We all use those two broad strategies to mask experience. Those mechanisms are our defenses. We're either focused on something else, tuned to a different station as it were, which pushes the pain or whatever into a shadowy background, or we're doing something very noisy, numbing our bodies and minds. The barriers to sensitivity are noise and distraction. In order to reach beliefs, memories, and feelings at a level of experience difficult to tolerate, the therapist simply helps the client become more sensitive. Of course one can be relaxed without processing anything, but not if you freely allow experiences to emerge and you stay with them. High sensitivity and an openness to experience lead quite naturally to the emotional and spiritual growing we have left to do. The sensitivity cycle is a way of increasing sensitivity for just that purpose.

The Stages

The cycle is composed of four stages, with a barrier at each stage.

STAGES	BARRIERS
relax, reorient	completion
clarity	insight
effective action	response
satisfaction	nourishment

First, there's a place where one relaxes, where one drops external concerns and allow your mind and body to reorient. This stage is a completion of one thing and an opening to what's next, allowing the next thing that wants to happen to come into consciousness. This step is passive and open to organic need. For example, say you've been working all day. You stop, relax and begin to realize you're hungry as hell. It's simply a matter of completing what you're doing and allowing the next need, or the next piece of unfinished business, to emerge into consciousness. On the other hand, to keep certain experiences from arising, like hunger or loneliness or pain, people often simply keep some activity from completing. They fixate on something, avoiding the relaxation and reorientation in which the painful experience would emerge. That kind of avoidance is called a completion barrier.

If one does complete and relax, a new experience emerges. And if we keep our awareness on this new experience long enough, it clarifies. We get clarity. Sometimes this clarity comes suddenly, after a period of confusion. It comes in the form of **insight**. Just like hunger emerging after a job is done, the person might next realize, "what I want is a tuna sandwich." If one is sensitive enough and stays long enough with an more and more precise experiences unfold. It is not just hunger, it is exactly what one wants to eat. (The sensitivity cycle applies as much to knowing what to eat or how to stand and move as it does to emotional processing.) One stays long enough to gather enough information to clarify experience. There's not really much work involved in that; as with meditation, it's just a matter of staying with it, keeping the channel open. Still, it's a deliberate openness, a willed openness, an observing and a taking in. One of the big things that makes psychotherapy work is all the techniques we use to help people stay in their experience. Time automatically clarifies and enhances. As one stays with an experience, it yields more and more information and builds towards insight and understanding. Habits that avoid gathering information and reaching clarity are called **insight barriers**.

Once the situation is clear, the person is ready to make some **response** to it, to take some kind of action. If he has allowed the situation to clarify, his actions will be more effective. If he is clear he won't go off and buy pizza pie when he wants miso soup. He won't make dumb mistakes. His responses will line up with reality. His responses will be effective and efficient, accurate, not wasteful. No blind alleys. Habits that avoid responding in this deliberate, conscious way are called **response barriers**.

When one is clear about needs and wants, actions are much more effective and efficient. They get better results, more **nourishment** and satisfaction. They get more of what one wants and needs. Habits that prevent taking in what is needed are called **nourishment barriers**. Getting what one needs, in turn, allows one to relax more. When a person finally gets what he needs, there's a big sigh. He yields up his efforts and relaxes. Then he completes the actions that satisfied the need. That is called coming to **completion**. Habits that avoid completion are **completion barriers**. With completion, one reorients, relaxes even more and gets more clarity, then a little more effectiveness, then a little more nourishment, and around and around. Over the full range of the cycle, clarity becomes wisdom, effectiveness becomes mastery and complete confidence, nourishment and satisfaction become bliss and fulfillment, and relaxation becomes deep, inner peace. The cycle can be a lifetime's endeavor or the actions of a moment.

The Barriers and Character Process

The insight barrier is about blocking incoming information. It can be blocked at the sensory level all the way up to the level of understanding or insight. There are people who avoid seeing certain things about themselves or about the world. This is particularly true of people in a sensitive-analytic character process. For them, there are truths too painful to remember or to face. Some experiences have been overwhelming for them, like severe child abuse, and they don't want those experiences to enter consciousness. What they learned from such experiences is that life is harsh and full of menace, and though they may not remember the experiences, the "fact" that life is full of menace is written all over them.

As a result, people with insight barriers experience an overall withdrawal from contact with others and with their own bodily experience. At the insight barrier, they are avoiding images, memories, situations, and/or thoughts that could bring painful or even terrifying feelings and realizations. So, they block seeing, feeling, knowing, understanding and contact. They look away. Typically, under emotional stress, they will have their hands over their eyes or they'll squeeze their eyes shut. They may have eye problems. Often they are people who focus themselves completely on something very unemotional, like computers. They often prefer to work by themselves, away from other people. Contact with others is difficult for them, clumsy. They are shy and easily embarrassed. Their preference, like Sheldon's ectomorphs whose shape they seem to favor, is for low lights, small rooms and closed doors. In the decade of the eighty's, some of them wear earphones all day with the music up loud. "No incoming calls," as my friend Louis Peacock used to say. Though they block sensory experience as part of this whole process, it is basically the meaning of their experience they are avoiding. They don't want to remember and recognize how unloved, unwanted or beaten they were. It seems that in a study of over a thousand cases of MPD, multiple personality disorder, the common history was severe child abuse. (Reported in *The Three-Pound Universe*, by Hooper and Teresi.)

When working with people at the insight barrier, you help them shut out the painful memory and make it okay to do so, until they are ready to see it and understand it. And when they are ready, you make it as bearable and as safe as possible for them to give up fighting with those realizations and to absorb and integrate them. When that long fight is over, they are finally free to know themselves, to let themselves be here in this world, in touch with the physical emotional reality of both themselves and others. They learn to look you in the eye, to be comfortable here.

You can be open to information and insight and still block at the next stage — taking action, making some kind of response. This is the response barrier. There are people who get this injunction early: "it better not be your fault!" They were blamed and made to feel guilty early on. Their best response was no response. They learned that it is easier and wiser just to wait out the storm. They became experts at delaying and at bearing up. These kinds of habits are part of the burdened-enduring character process. People in this process have strong response barriers: their habits are such that they have great difficulty responding. They feel they want to respond, but can't. Actually, another part of them doesn't want the responsibility. For them, the role of victim works. Frustrating and defeating other's people's purposes is the only victory they can imagine. Their own purposes don't seem to occur to them. Their responses and their responsibility get shoved under the rug.

These people bog down very easily. If you push them, they turn into rocks. The task, therapeutically, is to make it safe to respond. I avoid trying to get them to do anything. Rather, I help them hold back; in fact, I may physically hold them back while they mobilize that part of themselves that wants to move freely. In that way, I make it safe for them to express themselves. That helps them realize that they want to move and express, and to know a little bit of what it feels like. It's a taste of freedom and it is part of the knowledge that it's worth the responsibility that goes with it.

Next on the cycle is the nourishment barrier. Some people habitually push away available support and nourishment. Though it is dearly wanted, they're afraid it will soon be taken away. They're also afraid of their wanting. They are frightened by an image of a bleak future where they are alone, without strength, help, love, friends, or means. This drives them strongly to want all kinds of support and reassurances about support, which they refuse because it's too scary to accept it or believe in it.

That terrible conflict is the main ingredient of the dependent-endearing process. The long-term result is depression. The habit of disbelieving and refusing nourishment leads to weakness and collapse on the emotional level, just as the same refusal on the physical level would lead to physical collapse and death. You can offer nourishment to these people, but they won't take it in. They believe you are going to take it away again and that that experience will be too painful. They think that they'll only have what they need and want for a short while. They don't really trust you to continue with your giving. They doubt your sincerity. Their thoughts are locked on to ideas of deprivation and poverty.

With these people I work on taking in and using what's available. I help them see the cycle they're caught in and I give them only as much nourishment as they can believe in. It's a little at a time, so they can get used to it, as with a person breaking a long fast. I also help them learn, in Blake's beautiful words, to "kiss the joy as it flies."

Finally, there's the completion barrier, which is part of the industrious-overfocused or rigid process. Here, the difficulty is in letting go, letting *anything* go. Whether ideas or plans, situations, thoughts, relationships, tasks, loyalties, whatever, people with a rigid process have trouble letting these things complete. These people were rewarded for persistence, including both the external rewards of parents and the internal rewards of a boost of self-esteem. They did not get the simple love that parents were meant to give their children, the kind of love that builds a strong base of self-worth independent of performance. So, they know how to avoid emotions and relationships by just keeping busy with something else.

This process is closely tied to the metabolic effects of sympathetic enervation. It is a locking in of action and focus. People in this process have great difficulty relaxing. They want to look everything over one more time. They want to make sure. They want to go back to the house and see if they locked all the windows. They're list makers. Traditionally, they're called, obsessive-compulsives. It is hard for them to relax and re-orient, to give up one project and let another just come along. They stay busy. When the emotions become too strong for them, they take refuge in action. By being busy and mobilized and focused, they avoid feeling more of their needs and wants and pain.

With rigid processes, I try to avoid getting mobilized along with them and turning the therapy session into a search for solutions to problems. It is the mobilization itself which is the problem. If these people felt okay about themselves, they could relax and enjoy life, without the drive towards that "great accomplishment" that will finally earn them the love that was their birthright. With these people, I teach them to relax, allowing the heart to open, in the faith that it will be lovingly received. I help them find a self-worth that does not need performance. I help them complete the long frustrated search for a parent's love that had some all too human limit.

Feldenkrais' work has a lot to do with sensitivity. He teaches people (some with palsy-like symptoms) to move effectively. He teaches them to use arms that have never have been able to, to bring a glass of water to a thirsty mouth. Many people get lost trying to understand Feldenkrais' work because, ultimately, it seems too simple. He was not just using awareness to study movement; he was using movement to create awareness. He was creating a more precise body image, an awareness of the body that makes precise movement possible. At first, he made the movement for the person, over and over again. He moved the arm. He showed the person that first you have to do this and then you have to do this and then you have to move the shoulder, and so on. He didn't tell the person in words; he told the nervous system through the experience of the movement. He took the person piece by piece through the movement. He did it twenty or thirty times, sometimes fifty, until the movement came into that person's awareness. When it becomes aware, then it can be done. Awareness studies movement, movement creates awareness. There's this kind of mutuality in all organic systems.

According to Moshe, some of these people with the palsy-like symptoms never got a clear image of what a precise, easy arm movement is like because they could never repeat the movement enough times to create a clear image of it in the nervous system. So they couldn't get the awareness. The arm would go one direction one time and elsewhere the next. It was never consistent enough. There was too much noise in the system to get a clear signal. So they never got a chance to learn the movement. The shaking and the clumsy effort are movements full of noise. He says it takes about twenty careful repetitions to get a new movement into awareness and make it voluntary. The cerebral palsy people never got twenty in a row. So Feldenkrais gives them twenty in a row. And sure enough, they learn it. They become aware enough, they feel it, and they can do it. When they know clearly what it feels like, they can do it. It's both awareness through movement and movement through awareness. It's beautiful, the awesome power of mutuality.

There's no way to improve without that feedback. If you can't see how you're doing and how well you're doing, you're not going to get any better. To be mindful is to use feedback, to pay attention, to become masterful at living, to find harmony with your environment.

Sometimes, I sit in a hot tub, outside, on a cold day. Soaking in the steamy water with the jacuzzi going, I get my nose down into the water so my eyes are looking right out across the surface. Then, I watch the bubbles breaking. Every bubble that breaks sends a tiny droplet of water into the cold air. And every droplet invariably travels along a parabolic path. Billions of bubbles popping out of hot tubs the world over and always a parabola. Each one, leaping heavenward and falling back.

I'm reminded of the poem by Robert Frost, called, "The Silken Tent". One line talks about "its central cedar pole, which is its pinnacle to heavenward and signifies the sureness of the soul." This morning I was meditating, and, after a while, I could feel that direction in my body, that organizing of the system heavenward. And I realized: there is that impulse, that tendency, that reaching upward. We're trying to get there. We're are not perfectly vertical yet. We still fold up a lot, from pressure and fear. But we're heading in that direction. It's our nature, part of our love affair with gravity. And the falling back....

Death, said Gregory Bateson, is the way the species updates its files. It is a clearing out and a fresh start. The death of one is nature's way of making space to try another. The species is playing that game, not the individual. So, death is a completion and a reorientation, as childhood was a gathering of information and insight, as maturity is responsibility and effective action. Hopefully, the closing years will be filled with the satisfying rewards of a life lived consciously.

16

THE HABITUAL INTERRUPTION
OF EXPERIENCE:
BARRIERS AND CHARACTER

At each stage in the sensitivity cycle, there are ways to block further increases in sensitivity. When these ways become habitual, we call them barriers. The barriers interrupt the process of going deeper into experience. The sensitivity cycle is a process and the barriers are its interruptions. Habits at the barriers interfere with the natural unfolding of the cycle. At the completion barrier, habits prevent the completion of one process and the reorientation towards the next. At the insight barrier, habits block the taking in of information. Some people have things they don't want to see or understand. They prefer to be out of contact. They won't look at you. Under stress, they get confused, they withdraw. They avoid clarity. If they try to relax, they get numb. There is within their experience something too terrible to know. They may think there's something about them that's horrible. As a result, they avoid real contact with both what is within and what is outside. It leaves them very little room in which to live.

Other people see clearly, or somewhat clearly, but have habits that prevent action. They feel stuck, bogged down, heavy, thick and immobile. And hopeless. It feels to them as if there's nothing they can do about it. As impulses arise, an inner voice says, No! Don't do it! You might hurt somebody! You'll make another mistake. These habitual injunctions destroy all sense of fun and spontaneity. As impulses build up, people at this barrier tighten down on themselves. They brace themselves. The more you push them, the less willing they are to respond. The only way to assert themselves as children, to use the strength they had to live, or to protect their spirits, was to resist. So they are stuck in a pattern of: I am only true to myself when I resist or do nothing. You can't get anywhere with them using force. Any hint of your wanting them to do something automatically shuts them down. They cannot respond any other way to the perception of force or responsibility.

Then, there are people who commit to the lonely path of doing it all themselves. They don't expect any consistent support. They don't expect any real help from the outside. They don't expect nourishment. They have a view of the world as an empty place, where you can't count on anybody. When you offer nourishment, they reject it. They see something wrong with it. They won't take it in. As a result, they are never satisfied. They avoid taking in nourishment or even finding it in the world, because they do not want to deal with the possibility of loss. The state of getting what you want is anxiety producing. Having the thing so wanted leaves one vulnerable to loosing it again. They're not good at taking in what's available.

Lastly, there are those who stick with their actions long after they might stop and rest and wait for a new situation to emerge. As habit, this process interrupts spontaneity and maintains control. It also prevents any increase in sensitivity by keeping psychological and physical tension going. They view the world as problems to be solved through energy and effort and a place where love and affection are given only for achievement.

One way of working is to keep moving around the sensitivity cycle, increasing sensitivity and getting to experience. The therapist is trying to evoke insight, helping the person relax, providing nourishment of some kind, or supporting expression. At the response barrier, the issues are safety and responsibility. The therapist works to make it safe to respond, either by supporting expression and risk taking or by slowing things down, and making actions deliberate and real. At the insight barrier the job is to make contact. At the nourishment barrier, I help people explore the reactions to offers of nourishment. I help people understand that they are shutting out the very nourishment that they want the most. Then I help them learn to go past their fears and take nourishment in. At the completion barrier, I teach people to let go. I help them melt into receptivity and the relaxation of doing. All techniques at the barriers are parts of therapeutic strategy, different ways of dealing with the different character processes.

There are several ways to think about the barriers. They can often be indicators of core material and character processes. Each character process[1], with its own specific kind of core material, tends to organize behavior in particular ways, around particular dispositions and strengths. The interruptions of sensitivity are different in the different processes. As therapy moves through the various stages, the difficulties encountered, with contact or accessing for example, are signs of the particular character process operating. There is a connection for example between contact problems and the sensitive-withdrawn process, between accessing mindfulness, and the burdened-enduring and deceptive processes; between a barrier to nourishment and the dependent-endearing process, and completion and expressive and industrious processes. It's not so much that each character process uses just one barrier, but that the various processes use each barrier differently and are seen most clearly at only one or two of these barriers.

Each barrier also involves the balance of opposing tendencies. For example, at the insight barrier, the balance of contact and withdrawal. As a principle of organization, the balancing of opposites is one of the most used in nature. Some examples are the two sexes, the sympathetic and parasympathetic branches of the nervous system, and positively and negatively charged particles of the atom. This dynamic interplay of opposites is a prime mover and energizer of the universe. Figure and ground define, reveal and give life to each other. Perhaps its most beautiful representation is the yin-yang symbol. The failure to smoothly integrate any of the life central functions means that they will act in conflicting ways, just as the failure of a traffic light leaves a busy intersection snarled or hazardous.

The person with strong conflicts has a disposition towards one way of acting, which is to say they react rather than respond. A disposition to withdraw is part of the sensitive-withdrawn process. Impulsivity, quickness of reaction, is characteristic of the deceptive process and the opposite disposition, to delay, is a part of the burdened-enduring process. Barrier behaviors are painful, damaging, extreme and persistent. Unintegrated functions have a way of going off to one extreme and staying there. For instance, the withdrawal of the sensitive-withdrawn process leaves the person both desperate to make contact and out of touch with the information needed to do so with any chance of success. The results are abortive or inappropriate attempts to reach out, leading quite naturally to frequent failure, hurt and more reasons to withdraw. Each barrier shows these cycles.

The barriers then serve as defenses against hurt, separation, loss, failure and so on. By keeping sensitivity low and by re-directing behavior away from painfully charged areas, the barriers protect us. They do so first when we're highly vulnerable as children, then later, when as adults we have grown accustomed to being more or less out of touch with ourselves.

The Insight Barrier

The birth experience and the quality of contact with the mother and the environment in the earliest days, weeks and months are central. For the infant, there is no symbolic content; that comes later. The world is sensation and feeling.

If that world is unpleasant or painful, the infant will shrink from it by shutting down as well as it can. Only the mother's sensitivity to what is too much for the newborn, keeping it warm and dry and away from sudden noises, bright lights, etc, will allow the infant time to integrate in the world. If the mother is fearful, anxious, violent or too insensitive, the chances are that an insight barrier pattern will develop. On the other hand, the need for too much contact is also a possibility. The mother is more usually the safest, warmest, most attractive place of all to the child, and any separation from her can be extremely painful. Eventually the child learns to integrate this strong need with the development of an autonomous self. Failure of this development is the seed configuration for the expressive-clinging process.

These are the organizing factors of the insight barrier. If contact is harsh, the infant develops a tendency to withdraw. What options does the infant have? It can't walk out. It has to withdraw attention, shut down the senses. It cannot understand or ask you to change. It has only feelings and reactions. Once a pattern of withdrawal is set, the child organizes all subsequent learning around that pattern. If contact is overly important and separation is feared, the infant learns to control contact with clinging and distress.

Insight barrier behavior is a turning away, breaking or not making contact, fixating on something non-threatening. The tight, tense musculature of the sensitive-withdrawn is the physical aspect of withdrawal, both as a holding in of impulses and a way to create internal noise to drown out the harshness outside. It is this lack of contact with self and world as experience that is the core of the sensitive-withdrawn process. In contrast, many people who have sensitive-withdrawn dispositions or strategies are uncommonly good at understanding the world symbolically, especially within some narrow area of interest. The expressive-clinging person creates "emotional noise" to avoid breaking contact. Both processes are about distancing. The sensitive-withdrawn is trying to maintain a safe distance by withdrawing. The expressive-clinging feels safe only when there is little or no distance and no threat of separation. Anxiety in the expressive-clinging process is about some unwanted realization, pressing for awareness. All the strong feelings, the laughing and crying, are an attempt to avoid a realization that's all too close. Like the going out of contact of the sensitive-withdrawn, it blocks insight. Gathering information is the Life Central Function. In the sensitive-withdrawn, withdrawal and the breaking of contact disrupts the gathering of information about present, ongoing experience. Contact with the here and now is tenuous in the sensitive-withdrawn. Pieces of the conversation and information about what is going on right here and now are often lost.

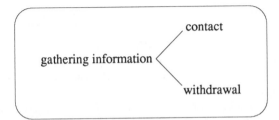

In the expressive-clinging, strong connections are made on the emotional and physical levels. The lack of distance, however, leaves little room to understand the situation. Distortion results. The ideal is fluid movement over the entire distancing function, from close, feelingful experiences to the concentration and abstract beauty of world-class chess or mathematics. The expressive-clinging process involves a desperation for closeness which tends to overwhelm and drive intimate others away. When others do stay, they feel trapped, pressured, manipulated, and so forth. This need of the other for distance is sensed easily by the expressive-clinging and creates emotional turmoil and even more desperation. Round and round.

In the expressive-clinging process, the pain of separation is often converted into high emotions, which are then used as part of the expressive-clinging production, itself designed to maintain contact. This tends to confuse the issue and leave it unresolved. It is the issue, sometimes framed in terms of being loved and needing love, that is clouded and avoided. Feelings are certainly present. They are not defended against. In fact, people who find this way of behaving easy are those who can make big feelings out of very little events. In contrast to most people, who defend against hurt by shutting down feelings, expressives are "amplifiers." It is the realization that the other needs distance that they defend against. The insight barrier, in both cases, is an adjustment to information that would overwhelm.

I worked with a woman in Portland, Oregon once who had the habit of asking a question and while I was answering it her head would turn and her eyes would go off into space. After I finished my answer she would turn back with a totally blank look. It was just as if I hadn't said anything and she hadn't asked the question. As a result, nothing seemed to work. Of course not, because we never connected. This is the flavor of insight barrier stuff. It took me a while, over an hour actually, to find something I could do with that. I had two assistants present. I decided to go directly for the barrier behavior. I thought we could take over the turning of her head and her not listening and see what happened. I set up a little experiment where she would to try to keep looking and listening to me as my assistants took over the tendency to turn away and the not listen. I explained the set-up to her. One assistant would put some physical pressure on her to get her head to turn away. The other assistant would whisper in her ear, "don't listen to him, don't listen to him." She would try to look and listen. We got set up and when she was ready, she signaled us and while one assistant whispered the words, the other was trying to move the woman's head away from looking at me. It only took a few seconds. Having shown very little emotion up till then, she suddenly broke down crying and got very emotional. We had taken over her contact avoidance technique, leaving her with the part of herself she was protecting, the part that hungered desperately for the contact she'd been avoiding. The first thing she remembered was being taken to an orphanage and being separated from her sister. The last felt need for contact with a loved one swept over her. That had been forty plus years before, when she'd been five. So, we processed the pain of that and the option of feeling and satisfying that need in her present and future life.

Working At The Insight Barrier

One way to work at the insight barrier is with the eyes. Just exploring the feelings and reactions created by looking at and looking away, if done with mindfulness, will generate a lot of material to work on. Being afraid of looking and being looked at is directly connected to core material. Much the same can be done with touch. The issue is contact and those are the two primary channels for it, Ma Bell not withstanding.

During an intensely emotional session, clients often want to fold up and be held tightly. This is an expression of the fear of falling apart if contact is made with the fearful thing. The sensation of being cold or frozen (in terror) is also part of it. If you hold the person very tight for a while, it will feel very comforting at first and after a while, many minutes at least, they may begin to feel the impulse to open. The person may spontaneously go into birth movements or experiences. This type of birthing process, besides being an intensely real experience and often directly related to the person's actual birth, it is the primary symbol of coming out, being here and making contact. After the person pushes out, she or he is ready to look at a face. This can be a fearful time for them. The first visual contact. It is also where the biggest change can take place, learning to look. Eyesight can even improve.

I always try to have a loving face waiting when those eyes finally open. I'll use an assistant or a member of the group, if it's a workshop. That face and the gentle touch and warmth of hands and skin are the original welcoming committee. For someone with a sensitive-withdrawn process, the experience of opening one's eyes after pushing out into the world and finding love waiting is like waking from a nightmare in the arms of a clear and loving parent.

In Albuquerque once, after I'd worked like this with a person in a sensitive-withdrawn process, the woman involved began noticing things, like colors or how pretty things were. We had worked in the late morning and all that afternoon she would suddenly see something and her face would brighten with wonder and delight. She'd be staring at something, a shadow maybe or the light on a tree outside and she would light up herself. She couldn't pay attention to class at all. She kept looking around; she hadn't known that things looked that way. I watched with great pleasure as she discovered her world.

Another thing I do at the insight barrier is to work on accepting inner impulses, making contact with the inner self, accepting the parts which are angry, fearful, whatever. The probes I use are about issues like belonging (you are welcome here) or fear (you don't have to see anything you're not ready to see). I also use probes like: :"you're human" or "whatever is inside you is natural." Such probes speak directly to the issues of withdrawn process.

The Response Barrier

The response barrier is about timing, control and the habits which mediate actions. Actions need to be timed, shaped and directed in order to be effective. For any action to be intentional, some time to plan it or think about it is needed. Intention requires deliberation, if only for a moment. Only if our actions are deliberate, can we feel responsible. Only when time and deliberation and consciousness shape action do we feel that we have done it; that it is our decision and we own our connection to the outcome. Then we are responsible. If we are free to act, able to respond or not, then we are responsible (response-able) for the action. If we are not free, if the action takes place suddenly, without our intention on any conscious level, if we only react or find ourselves unable to act, then we do not feel responsible. So, the response barrier has a lot to do with time.

Two character processes are closely involved with the response barrier, the burdened-enduring and the deceptive. Delaying tactics, stuckness, an inability to respond and the role of innocent victim are hallmarks of the burdened-enduring process. It is action controlled to the point of inaction. It is delay and procrastination to the point of failure. Fear of responsibility motivates that control. For burdened-enduring processes, delay and resistance are automatic. Any effort to move the burdened-enduring process along results in automatic resistance and further delay. The slow and grudging actions of those with safe, dull jobs comes to mind.

The deceptive process, on the other hand, is about resisting too little and taking action impulsively without thought or conscious planning. It ends up with the person acting irresponsibly and feeling not responsible at all. While the burdened-enduring plays at innocence and feels quite guilty, the deceptives play at responsibility and feel none of it. It's the deceptives who are impulsive, unreliable and glib. It's the deceptives who lay claim to talents, attributes, wealth, status and power for which there is little or no reality. The primary traits of the deceptives are a lack of commitment to the truth, which in another sense is just their unrestrained imaginations, and a near total lack of guilt. When one's actions are completely spontaneous and impulsive, responsibility is lost. David Shapiro talks about this idea in his book, *Autonomy and Rigid Character*.

Quick actions are mediated by sympathetic enervation and low cortical inhibition. The opposites of these, parasympathetic enervation and high cortical inhibition, mediate slow, deliberate action. So, these factors, metabolism and the inhibitory influences of the cortex, help set the patterns of behavior around the response barrier. In the stages where control of the voluntary muscles is being learned, where free movement is being experimented with, where rules are being given by the parents and tested by the child, the shape of action and responsibility is taking form. It is then that the burdened-enduring learns that delay and innocence will wear out one's oppressors and the deceptive-imaginative learns that breaking the rules can be gotten away with by means of lies told and charm. The swiftness of the deceptive-imaginative's excuses, disarming as they are, have much the same effect as the burdened-enduring's poor, bedraggled clumsiness. Each ends up not responsible

At the response barrier, the burdened process image is one of endurance, bearing up and waiting it out, like the turtle. Holding out, never giving in, these are the essential equipment of delay. Contrariwise, the image of freedom from the needs and wants of others, or the need to plan or take account, these are the cornerstones of impulsivity. Like Superman able to do anything, to help the needy, to rescue those in danger with no chance of failure, effortlessly, to fight the doers of evil, without any loss of one's infinite energy and no danger to oneself. These images of freedom and invulnerability are the symbolic foundation of response barrier behavior.

The polar aspects of impulse and control need to be integrated. Times are either serious, insignificant or in between. To hold off or jump in has to be decided for oneself and others. For the burdened-enduring, life is somber. For deceptives, it's all just a joke.

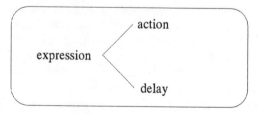

It isn't, couldn't be, serious. "I didn't mean it, guys. Just kidding. What's everyone so excited about? Okay, so I don't have a pilot's license. I meant to get one."

Response barrier behavior is an adjustment to control by others and a defense against the pain of separation from loved ones who, like parents, expect and often demand, a certain level of responsibility. At the response barrier, the disposition is either to delay, as in the burdened-enduring process, or to react without deliberation, as in the deceptive process. Delay makes others impatient. Claims to innocence make others want to force action and responsibility and to mete out punishment. Impatience and force directed at someone in a burdened-enduring process only further delays action and sets the stage for a long, silent battle of wills. The person in a deceptive process will answer with promises and charm and will try to still the demands of others with only a semblance of what's wanted, thus raising more demands and outcries about failing to do what's right and what's expected. The game goes on until the process blows up.

The Nourishment Barrier.

The three character processes associated with the nourishment barrier are the dependent-endearing, the self-reliant and the deceptive. The tendency to see less than really is there, to avoid wanting or expecting too much, this is nourishment barrier behavior. It is central to the dependent-endearing process. The tendency to go it alone, to do for oneself and the reluctance to accept support from others mark the self-reliant process. The deceptive-imaginative process person is often busy supporting others and being the nice guy or is doing something stupid and dangerous, not really taking the time to evaluate what's good for him or what he really needs.

The nourishment barrier is about taking in nourishment and avoiding things toxic. It's about evaluating the results of one's actions. In the dependent-endearing process it can be seen as a disposition to abort or collapse. The dependent-endearing's view of the world as barren makes everything look like a difficult struggle. An attitude like that fosters a disposition to abort all efforts and collapse when the going gets the least bit difficult. The tough may get going when the going gets tough, but those who are habitually dependent-endearing simply poop out. The disposition to evaluate the situation as unpromising stops them before they start. Self-reliants have more staying power. Theirs is a disposition to pursue lone challenges, a bias towards facing into the wind and a penchant for the constant testing of the self. It is a tendency to deny one's need for others, or for support and companionship.

Problems at the nourishment barrier effect ones ability to evaluate the results of one's actions. Much that could be supportive is found wanting and is dismissed.

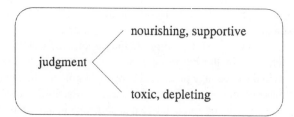

People in a depressed state have a knack of converting any potentially positive aspect of their situation into a terrible liability. If they inherit millions, they worry about the taxes. Such persons may also believe that they too have been judged and found wanting, the same evaluation turned inward. For the self-reliant, the support of others is not recognized or accepted. For the deceptive-imaginative, the toxic is unrecognized, all the way from doing too much for others and depleting oneself to defying seriously dangerous situations. For creatures like us, so dependent upon language and meaning, deception is a ruinous strategy. For chameleons it works. They don't think about who's a good guy and who isn't, who means them well and who is out to take them, who deserves their energies and who does not. For those judgments, you have to think a bit and you have to be able to see worth and danger in every place and person. The conflicts that surround these processes have to do with giving and taking, with reaching out for nourishment and support and denying the need for these.

The Completion Barrier

This last barrier is all about persistence and the problem of completion. After a person has taken in sufficient nourishment, the next thing to do is relax, rest and reorient. At completion, the system begins to reorganize its hierarchy of needs. As one need is fulfilled another emerges. Completion is a problem when the person doesn't reorient, doesn't allow a process to complete. The person might have trouble letting go of each small task or one central relationship. Like the guy who takes his work home, or the one who calls home ten times a day from the office. The completion barrier is about trouble letting go. One way this barrier is expressed is as a fear of being spontaneous. A person must relax control to be spontaneous. The habit here is to stay in control. The fear is that one will give up too soon. With a little more effort, one could make it. The style is to stick to it, try harder, give 110% and get it perfect. The people involved in completion barrier processes are trying to keep something going. They persist when others would relent. They push against their tiredness and hunger. Theirs is walking against the wind, the uphill battle, frustration and self-denial. The focus is on performance, not pleasure. Life is full of problems to be solved.

This barrier has to do with the failure to integrate letting go and persistence; control and passivity; the serious, hard work of adulthood and the play and magic of the child.

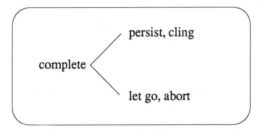

It is a failure to integrate the need for concentration and control with the need to let go, lay back and let nature take its course.

In going through the completion barrier, one goes from a sympathetic set to a parasympathetic set. It is a letting down, a relaxation. We expect soft feelings to emerge, tenderness, affection. The industrious-overfocused types have trouble softening and trouble with soft feelings like crying. They are pushing to be adults and they run from childish things. When they do let go, the child emerges. Therapy involves interactions centered on soft feelings. The disposition is to persist, to cling. Most people usually know when they have had enough of something, when it's time to quit and when it might pay to continue.

Notes for Chapter 16

1. Though terms like deceptive-imaginative or burdened-enduring are used occasionally throughout, they should always be understood to mean a person who uses these patterns habitually.

17

JUMPING OUT OF THE SYSTEM

You cannot be conscious of what you're not conscious of.

- Julian Jaynes, The Origin of Consciousness in the
Breakdown of the Bicameral Mind

There is no compassion without humor.

-- Da Free John, from a talk

---

*It is an inherent property of intelligence that it can jump out of
the task it is performing, and survey what it has done; it is
always looking for, and often finding patterns.*

— Douglas R. Hofstadter, Godel, Escher and Bach

G urdjieff called it sleep. We are not aware of our own processes. It is rare to find someone who really knows herself or himself. The patterns in our own behavior, the character patterns like sensitive-withdrawn and dependent-endearing are basically habits. They are habits of style, of thinking, feeling, doing, and being. And as habits they operate automatically and outside of awareness. For example, much of our internal dialog is repetitious, systematic and predictable. Someone said, we all talk to ourselves; we just don't listen. Our way of doing things is also repetitious and unconscious. These systematic aspects of ourselves are expressions of core material and appear in the therapeutic relationship as they do everywhere else. In therapy we use these patterns deliberately — to focus the process and to access the core material which motivates and shapes them. The systematic is grist for the therapeutic mill. Character is system; jumping out is freedom and autonomy.

Mental Doing

It is hard for the mind to be silent. I remember the first time I consciously experienced mental silence. I was meditating. Inside I was thinking: ah, it's quiet now. No it's not! I just said, it's quiet and no, it's not. And I said, I just said that. It went on and on. Every time I noticed a few seconds of silence I would break the silence to comment on it and then notice that I had commented. Only it didn't seem like me doing it. I was trying to be silent, damn it! I got so frustrated that spontaneously I screamed inside at all those voices, SHUT UP! And they did! For a little while, a minute maybe, it was perfectly, beautifully, peacefully silent. For me it was a revelation. I understood what was possible. No matter what else you achieve in this life, it will not equal that.

Mental silence, for most people is rare. Almost all the time we are busy inside, doing, planning, talking. If you spend even a few minutes casually studying what is going on in your mind, naming it, maybe writing it down, you'll find there's a pattern to all the activity. It has form and direction, pattern and purpose. It is *doing something.* You may be seeing pictures, creating fantasies, or acting out conversations and little dramas, or lecturing to yourself on some subject of interest (one of my favorites). Whatever it is, it is related to character patterns and the systems you are involved in. There may be an imagined or implied audience. For me, the fact that I'm lecturing (even to myself) sets up the role of teacher and the complimentary role of students. In my life I have had hundreds, if not thousands of people to whom I have related as a teacher to a student. The patterns of mental doing have a strong influence on how our lives unfold.

Mental doing serves to make us feel more secure in some way — it binds anxiety. As we talk to ourselves and watch the scenes we create, we are preparing, rehearsing, planning, or creating images and dramas in which we get something we need. Of course this internal activity can be overwhelmed and disintegrate when anxiety, worry or fear are too much. Still the goal of all this doing is some kind of satisfaction and it is related to core material and character.

Let's take a few examples. Suppose the mental doing jumps all over the place, never staying very long with one image, fantasy, dialog. The inner "audience" is always changing. This pattern could reflect a need to avoid staying too long or getting too close or taking on responsibilities. My lecturing for example, while it helps me prepare for some of the the realities of my life, it also keeps me in the position of authority and at some distance to my audience. In my case it is clearly a reflection of a tough-generous pattern. In the same way, internal fantasy and drama often reflect the clinging-expressive style. Mental doing serves character. Mental doing also draws others into recurring patterns of interaction with us. The underlying need is the same. We merely substitute an external audience for the internal one. Responses from the external world also help us to bind anxiety. So, we tend to draw real people into the roles we'd like them to play in our lives, just as we create imaginary people for our internal worlds. (Of course it isn't always this simple. There are also complimentary relationships between internal and external worlds and between conscious and unconscious. But the themes are still the same, the core material is the same.) Therapists, being in close, intimate relationships with others, can also be drawn into roles which serve the other's character needs. Hopefully, they will sense what's going on, discover it early, be able to name it for themselves and for the other and finally jump out of the system it has created.

Something about the other — the style, the role — draws the therapist into a systematic way of interacting. Using this perspective we can examine the character patterns in terms of what systematic tendencies they will exhibit, interacting with the therapist. The self-reliant for example has core material that organizes behavior around beliefs like, "I'm better off doing it myself" or "I don't expect anyone to help me." In therapy, people in this pattern will do most of the work themselves. They will listen to the therapist for a moment and go off somewhere inside their heads and work on it — whatever it was. When they come out, they will talk for a while and when the therapist responds, they go back inside and work some more, leaving the therapist pretty much twiddling her or his thumbs. I call that pattern of interaction with the therapist, pit stopping. It's like they are out there driving around the track and come in only rarely for some fuel or a tire change. It leaves the naive therapist feeling deflated or bored and thinking, what the hell am I doing here. A list of therapist client interactive systems is given below. First let's tackle the systems that therapists tend to bring to the work, especially those systems that disrupt the unfolding of the other's process.

Helping, Not Making

The system that we all slip into much too easily ignores the organicity of the other and assumes a power and control we have no right to. It is the system we all grew up in, the one that treats children as property and is held together by violence and threats to violence. It is reflected in therapy by therapists assuming that they have to do something, because the responsibility to make something happen rests with them. It is as if midwives felt responsible for making people pregnant and pushing babies out. Of course there are legitimate jobs for midwives and therapists, jobs like setting the environment and having knowledge of what to do when the unfolding process needs support and guidance. But the process is essentially organic and proceeds from within the other. Most therapists that I've noticed interfering with the other's unfolding process do it out of a need they have to *make* something happen, instead of knowing that they are there to *help* something happen.

In a very simple way, we see this system operating when therapists do not respond to what is already going on with the other (with a contact statement, for example), but attempt to force things along by experimenting too much and asking unnecessary questions; indulging their curiosity and their biases about where they want the process to go. The process has its own way to go. It is part of this system to look for what isn't happening — because it doesn't feel the aliveness of the other — rather than noticing what is happening. But noticing and naming the other's experience, especially the part that has present emotional content, is the response that best supports what is already unfolding. Naming and waiting for the other to decide where he or she will go from this present moment hands back responsibility and authority to the client. It is easy to do when you jump out of the authoritarian model, difficult when you don't.

A Short List

Now let's look at various systems that emerge that keep the unfolding process from evolving. First, the list, a few typical therapist-client interactive systems that come up in therapy and need jumping out of. Each of these systems — and this is only a small sample — is not just a troublesome way of interacting. Each is a reflection of core material. As therapist, recognizing that you are in something like this and finding a way to jump out of it is an essential step. Each system is a potential access route to the core material that organizes it. The following are all examples of something systematic in the behavior of the client. He or she:

1. Thinks about everything, analyzes a lot
2. Automatically delays, slows things down
3. Automatically disagrees
4. Re-words or refines everything the therapist says, translates everything the therapist says into his or her own language
5. Constantly asks questions
6. Does all of her or his own work, staying inside or simply talking without seeming to want or expect a reply
7. Can't or won't stay in present experience
8. Offers endless details and facts, no emotional content
9. Is intensely and continuously emotional
10. Dramatizes his or her situation extensively

11. Changes topics a lot
12. Wants therapist to direct
13. Doesn't volunteer anything, must always be lead
14. Does everything the therapist wants, even looks for what is wanted or expected, without seeming to ever have own needs, wants or agenda, tries to please the therapist

Jumping: The How and What

When we find ourselves in a system, we jump out in a very simple and direct way: we **shift the focus of the attention to the system itself**. We change the subject. We interrupt the ongoing content and name the system. Here's a couple of examples:

T: You know, I notice that you do a lot of thinking and I don't see any feelings.
C: Yes, I guess I do. My whole life is like that.
T: Is it okay with you if we look at that?
C: Sure.
T: Okay, let's do a probe. (The therapist then does a probe like: It's okay to feel. Or, whatever you feel is okay. Something like that.)

Second example:

T: I notice that you re-word everything I say. I imagine as a child they didn't let you have your own reality. (Often the case.)
C: (Gets immediately emotional.) No, they didn't. (In an emotional, slightly childlike voice.)
T: (Switches to working with the child — a gentle, slow, caring voice.) Well, I can understand why that makes you so sad and angry.
C: (A definite shift to looking like a crushed child.)
T: So, you're feeling pretty bad, huh. You needed someone to really believe in you, didn't you.
C: (Nods.)
T: That's really important isn't it?

And on into working with the child. In each of these examples, the therapist, jumps to a different level of interaction. It's not just jumping around from one aspect of the content to another. It's leaving the content to focus on the style, the context, the way the content is being presented. Within an established helping relationship, such interruptions are easily accepted. When the shift is to something highly significant for the other, the transition to the new focus is surprisingly easy and usually fruitful.

The jumps we make in therapy are from content to form, from statement to assumption, from surface structure to experiential base, from experience to meaning, from what we're doing to who's doing it and how, from thought to thinker, from piece to pattern, from character to core. Character is the mechanical in us. It is habit and pattern and unconscious structure, a mindless repetition of a way of doing everything, based on images and beliefs that rarely reach the surface. Attention, awareness and mindfulness are jumping power. To the extent that we are mindful, we can see the mechanical and that's the first step towards change.

In therapy, we notice things that are out of awareness for the client. It's not so much that this material is repressed; it's just habit. We notice say, a tone of voice. We draw attention to it: "You sound like you're not sure I'll believe you." We notice an habitual gesture or facial expression: "Are you aware of how you're moving your hands each time you talk about yourself?" Jumping, out of the content and into some part of the larger picture. It involves going from one level of a process, with one set of constraints, to a higher level, with fewer constraints. It is going from talking about something to noticing the way you're talking about it. It is going from being in some pattern of behavior, to noticing the pattern.

Imagine: you fall asleep in your favorite chair and you're dreaming. You're in a tower room. You're looking at a painting of a forest scene. You're in the forest. In the forest you have no awareness of being in a painting, a tower, a dream, asleep, in your favorite chair. You are embedded several levels below conscious awareness. As you start jumping out you first feel the two dimensionality of the trees around you and realize you're looking at a painting. You're back in the tower room, you see the painting for what it is. You walk to the tower window and look out over the town. You see the bells in the church steeple swinging. The sound reaches you and you begin to awaken. Then it's clear you were dreaming and the old clock on the wall has been chiming the hour. You've jumped out of the dream into your waking life.

The terrible compulsion of character patterns, all thick moods, tense boundaries and mysterious sources. How like dreaming it all seems.

It's the therapist's job to detect the systems of character operating and to help the client jump out of them. If this reminds you of art and philosophy, it should. If it reminds you of mindfulness and meditation, good! Art, philosophy, the growth of culture, science, literature, they're full of jumps from one level of understanding to another. From specific theories to general ones. From Newtonian physics to quantum theory and relativity. From physics to metaphysics, communication to meta-communication From Roman numerals to the decimal system, from algebra to calculus, from something simple to something more complex. From habit to conscious choice, from mechanical to organic, from "cause and effect" to feedback loops, from ego to freedom.

Listen to Da Free John: "There is no compassion without humor. No love without pleasure. No freedom without enlightenment."

Hofstaedter says the difference between humans and machines is that machines don't get bored. Humans get bored, tired of the same old patterns. And we have the imagination to jump out. In humor, poetry, art, mathematics, in all that requires imagining, we are the best. We are the grand jumpers of the planet earth — higher, wider and quicker. What other animal could reach the moon? Nobody's cow, that's for sure. Not even those wonderful birds that fly the full circle earth, whose kind have flown it for a million of years. Not even them. Just us. To the damn moon! What a jump it was.

As history attests, even that super jumping machine, the collective human mind, gets stuck. And individual minds are even more susceptible. Jumping, though it is our birthright, takes practice and a will.

Gift and Loss. Imagination also plays a big part in the painful patterns we get stuck in. In Kurt Vonnegut's novel *The Breakfast of Champions*, the protagonist is daily getting more crazy. His fellow towns-people however, the waitresses, the gas station attendants, the people who work for him and see him every day, they all fail to notice. They don't see him going nuts because they don't see him at all. In Vonnegut's words, they see their "expectations of him." They are merely imagining him as they've always known him. He's fixed somehow in their minds. Using clues like tone of voice, clothes, walk or whatever, they identify him and fill in all the rest with their imaginations. Vonnegut calls imagination, "the flywheel on the ramshackle machinery of the awful truth."

It is the great gift. Its dark side hides a terrible loss. If we mostly imagine the people around us, not really seeing them, not truly feeling them, we lose an immense world. We lose contact with what simply is. We lose the intensity of childhood. We lose magic and myth and get lost in the words and pictures of our minds. The mystic tries to go beyond them. The scholar, to be their master, not their slave. When they succeed they're free, to be who they truly are, to experience the world fully, to enjoy both its meaning and its mystery.

We're both free and stuck. In our stuckness, we end up seeing only our expectations. We get used to each other. We act on bits and pieces, a word, a gesture, mere clues. We go on being with each other without really seeing or knowing. It's not just the new haircut we miss, or age creeping up. We miss the experiences the other is living and the meaning they have. In the trance of ordinary consciousness, in the ceaseless chatter of the mind, we are constantly losing one another. It's this we have to jump out of. As Bhagwan Shree Rajneesh once put it, "while I am talking, you can be arguing with me in your head, thinking, questioning. But while you do, you are missing me. I am a fact here! You need not dream here." — We are all facts here.

It's the therapist who makes therapy come alive — by really being here alive and awake to what is happening in this very moment. It's not just bits and pieces to move the hour along. It's not just labeling and making symbols of one another and interacting with that. All too often the process goes from the freshness of a first encounter to a dull, stale ritual. That seems the normal course of things. We sink into the rituals of hello, how are you, no real answer expected. We think it is natural for the real person to fade from sight, to be replaced by habit and familiarity. It's hard work to keep each other fresh in our minds and hearts, to keep jumping out of the trance and into something live and real. But it's easier and a lot more fun than work. Anyway, it's what we're paid for.

Humor is often a jumping out. A little story. I used to live with a guy named Eliot. I was just starting out as a therapist and El was a student at the local college. He couldn't afford real therapy, so he tried to do it on himself. *Tried* is the operative word here. Eliot was a rigid guy and, well.... One afternoon, I was lying on my bed watching TV (football or something), with my door open, and El was in his room, with his door open, and he was trying to do bioenergetics on himself! He was trying to get a spontaneous release. Trying! Naturally, he was just getting frustrated. Because, as any school kid or Zen master knows, you can't make the spontaneous happen. Eliot was tying himself in knots. He'd scream a little, but that was forced and didn't offer any real release. So he'd get frustrated and try harder. And so on and on, into the afternoon...

Well, I wasn't going to close my door. First of all, I would have to get up off the bed to do that. And second, I thought Eliot ought to close his door, but I wasn't going to tell him that. I was just going to lie there and get more and more sullen. So I was fuming inside when ol' El finally dragged what was left of himself into my room. He sat dejectedly on my bed, his head hanging, and a small, weak voice he said to me, "I'm really frightened, Ron, I can't eat my supper." (El wanted some sympathy and I was ready to have him for my supper.) Well, I turned to look at him. He still had his head down, looking at his knees. He didn't look frightened at all. He looked and sounded like a big mope to me. I wasn't feeling the least sympathetic. After a moment, I just took a breath and cranked up the Voice of Maximum Compassion. Then, in that soft, slow, loving voice, I told him,

"Don't worry, Eliot. I'll eat your supper." A quiet moment went by, after which his head came up, and with a genuinely puzzled look on his face, he asked me,

"What did you say?" Apparently, my answer wasn't among the possibilities he'd been entertaining. So, I repeated my kind offer. And he broke out laughing. He laughed so much he just fell into my arms. After a while he went to eat his supper and I went back to the TV, a little bit appeased.

I love humor in therapy — to jump out of heavy, sad, unnecessary moods, to laugh at foolishness, my own as well as yours. I like to imagine I'm up on the heights sometimes, seeing the big picture, full of compassion and a big belly laugh.

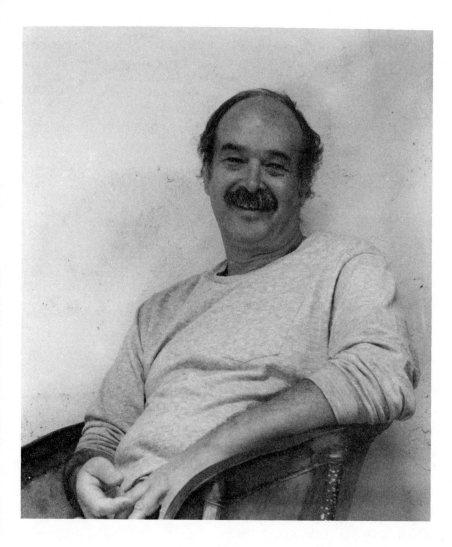

EPILOGUE

There's always more to say, more discoveries that seem important — and are important. There is always something new, something bigger than I can yet grasp. So, this ending is not really an ending for me; it is only a pause, a chance to rest and catch my breath. I wrote this book over a period of ten years. I learned as I went along. I learned what I did by experiment and inspiration. I learned it in the company of students, colleagues, workshop participants and clients. I had a living laboratory. I had time and an unflagging desire to study. In those ten years, I have seen the Hakomi Institute grow from an idea into trainings in eighteen cities, on two continents, with over twenty active teachers and hundreds of students. I think this growth will continue, for this reason: it is a part of the growth of consciousness that's taking place everywhere.

It may help to take one last look at this global change, to feel its qualities and sense its meaning. First, there are new models in science. The book, *Turbulent Mirror*, by John Peat and F. David Biggs, tells beautifully how our view of reality is changing. The real world is a much more complex, dynamic world than we formally believed. It is fluid and self-organizing. There is a wholeness and an interconnectedness we didn't recognize before. The world is alive in both a new and an ancient sense. I believe this aliveness will be recognized, nurtured and fiercely defended in the days to come. People will claim this aliveness as their birthright. It will become the cornerstone of teaching, morality and international relations. The new model is a better tool for dealing with our world and those who embrace it will inherit its power. They will be better able to understand and participate in every aspect of living. The deadness of the old models is a deadness of feeling, a crushing incapacity to experience. It allows us to exploit the weak, to war in our hearts and to condone the beating of children. Violence devastates the true self in both perpetrator and its victim. The new model makers, like family systems psychologist and teacher, John Bradshaw, make this terrible truth all too clear.

Second, we are in a revolution. It is a revolution in how we know and relate to ourselves, each other and the world around us. Like all revolutions, it is a combination of hope and desperation. The hope is that we will grasp these new ways and bring a fruitful peace to the whole planet. The desperation is: we haven't much time. The old ways are killing us. It's not so different from psychotherapy — a mixture of deadness and hope for change.

I see the work I've helped create going out on its own now, like a grown child leaving home. It is strong and sure in its own right. There's less chance to fool with it, changing things. Other trainers, each his or her own expression of the principles, are teaching their own students, now. As I let it go, I hope I've made this child strong and healthy. I hope it will do well. In a way, I'm glad this phase is over. My life will be easier, my mind, quieter. I'll look to family — my wife Terry and my newborn daughter, Lily. I'll be working more on training materials. There will always be new things to study, new books to write.

HOW I KNEW ...

I'd like to to tell you about how I knew God wanted me to be a psychotherapist. It has to do with a guy who was breathing a certain way.

I'd never done psychotherapy. I'd been in encounter groups and stuff like that on the West Coast. One time, after I'd been in therapy with Arthur Janov for two weeks and nothing happened, I was broke, I owed money and I was in a bad way. I was thinking of going back and getting my old job at the bowling alley or something equivalent. I was passing through Albany, New York. (You wouldn't think a man's whole life could change in Albany, N.Y.) I stopped there to spend a few days with an old friend of mine who was the staff psychologist at Albany Medical College. This man, who was a great lover of God, one of the true faith, a lover of Meher Baba, said to me, "Why don't you come up to the hospital and be a guest therapist?

As I said, I'd never done a lick of psychotherapy in my life, so I said, "Of course. Yes, I'll be glad to." Being a psychopath, I assumed I was a psychotherapist. (You can almost feel invisible hands at work already.) My first day there, my friend introduced me to a group of people from the locked ward and the staff, who were sitting around in a circle waiting for group psychotherapy. He introduced me as guest therapist. That's it. I'm on.

I looked slowly around at everybody. I was looking for where the energy was. I'd been in encounter groups and that's what you did, so I did it. You don't want to work unless there's energy around. So, I'm looking around, stopping to look at each person and I come to this one guy who's staring intently at me. I figure he's got it. He's got the energy. So I say to him, "I sense that you're angry. Is that right?"

He answers. In my whole life I never heard such a voice. This guy's voice sounds like it's coming out of an empty, fifty-gallon oil drum. It's totally hollow and deep. He says, "Yeaahs." Suddenly I realize... I'm in cuckoo land! I tell myself, "Go ahead anyway. What's to lose?"

So I ask him, "Would you like to work with that?"

Again, "Yeaahs." I decide I'll do what those encounter group guys do. I motion with my hand and tell him, "Why don't you lie down?" Then I look at the floor. It's linoleum. I want to get him kicking and banging but the floor's cold and hard. The staff and I talk about the floor for a minute till someone runs out and gets a rug, about one foot square. I'm not impressed by the rug but I am by the person's running out and getting one. These staff people have been in the hospital longer than the patients and they have heard that a new age is dawning and here's a guest therapist from the magical coast asking a patient, the first in the history of New York State, to lie on the damn floor. Worth watching? Worth running out for a rug? You bet!

The guy lies down on the little rug. I'm planning to get him kicking and banging and yelling. Get that angry stuff out. That's the policy. Well, first thing I notice is he is breathing backward. He tightens his stomach when he breathes in. So I figure I'd better fix that first, before we kick and bang. Now this is a room of maybe twenty patients on a locked mental ward in a big hospital with nurses, doctors, psychiatrists and residents, fifteen or so, all gathered around. I kneel down next to this guy on the floor. I get one hand on his belly and with the other, I stroke his head. I'm going to get him to breathe right and I'm using one hand to help him feel the movement in his belly and the other to soothe him.

I'm not thinking at all about how all this might look to these people who don't touch their patients and definitely don't get down on the floor with them. I imagine they were saying to themselves, "What kind of mumbo jumbo is this?" But I'm not thinking about that. I'm tripping gaily along thinking, "Isn't this nice, being a psychotherapist."

So, I'm leaning over this guy, whispering in his ear, nobody able to hear a word I'm saying, except me, and I guess him. I tell him, "Listen, try to get my hand to go up when you breathe in. Okay?" It takes about two minutes. Finally he gives a big sigh and starts breathing right. I say, "That's wonderful. That's right. Keep doing it." And he keeps sighing and doing it. After a while he's breathing nice and easy and I'm whispering encouragement. I feel like I'm on top of everything now. Except he isn't talking. He doesn't answer my questions. He hasn't said a word for three or four minutes now. In point of fact, he's asleep. He's sleeping! I want to say something like, "Are you awake?" but I'm afraid of what all these people will think. I'm supposed to be doing therapy and the patient has fallen asleep.

So I decide to get up, sit in my chair and look like I know what I'm doing. I figure that's my best shot. I get back in my seat with a look of confidence, as if to say, "This is what is supposed to happen, folks. I was going to get him to kick, but he fell asleep and he can't hear me anymore. Happens all the time." Confident, you know. Then I look back at him and see that he has peed all over the floor. He peed on the floor. I guess while we were down there together with me looking close at his eyes and whispering in his ear. And I never noticed it. There's a long silence. Believe me! I'm not going to say anything because I haven't the slightest idea what's going on. Beats me. They're not going to say anything either. Maybe they're figuring it's a new method — pee on the floor therapy. More likely they're wondering if they should let me out or not.

The long silence is broken when he cools off a bit and wakes up. He pops up on his elbows and looks around. Without saying anything he looks at steadily at me. Words simply fail me. I'm in shock. It could have ended right there, my whole career, I mean. Some nurse had the presence of mind to ask him if he wanted to go change his clothes. He nodded, yes and left the room silently. I'd been saved. I still think I'm in charge, so I ask, Any questions?" Give me a hint, right? I need some support here. The whole group, everybody, in one synchronized movement, turns slightly away from me. Their eyes keep looking at me, but their heads and bodies turn away. No questions. Not one. Thirty-five people in the room and none of them has a single thing they want to ask me. I figure, "That's it. I bombed. I don't need to be a psychotherapist. I'll be a writer." It's very quiet.

Right then he comes walking back in. Maybe he'll talk to me. He sits down and I say, "How are you doing?" And, in a perfectly normal voice, a beautiful, soft, full bodied voice, he says, "I feel wonderful." BOOM! An electric ripple goes though the people there. I can feel it. "Wow, look at that!" That's what they're thinking. "Look at that. How did that happen?" I'm back. They had been trying to turn this guy around for weeks and me, with my quiet confidence and magic hands did the job in fifteen minutes. Of course, I know — a little miracle has happened. If not in the patient's life, then certainly in mine. I begin to feel the angels around me. I imagine they have strict orders concerning my career development. I hear the commands coming down to them, "Get Kurtz out of there! Get him out!" Somebody up there, as the expression goes, wanted me to be a psychotherapist and He had bailed me out.

So, that's how I knew. I mean if He got me out of that one, He must want me to be a psychotherapist. So, I knew. Once in a while, after that fateful development, while I still lived in Albany, I'd run into the guy who headed the psychiatric part of the hospital. The first thing he'd always say was, "He's still out." He was referring to the guy who peed on the floor. The guy had gotten out of the hospital a week later and never got put back in. In fact he went around telling people how I'd saved him. Well, we know who saved who.

Sometime, I'll have to tell you the story of the next day when I tried to repeat myself and blew it completely. A real disaster. But that didn't effect my career. I was already sure I was going to be a psychotherapist.

Appendix
Outline of Method and Techniques

1. establishing a healing relationship **(techniques:** tracking, contact and acknowledging)
2. development and deepening of access routes
   a. spontaneous emergence **(techniques:** joots, contact, acknowledging)
   b. lowering the noise **(techniques:** support, safety and nourishment)
   c. deliberate evocation: **(general techniques:** deepening and meaning questions, suggestion of passivity)

   1. beliefs **(technique:** probes)
   2. feelings:
      fear **(techniques:** take over management, search for safety)
      sadness **(techniques:** meaning questions)
      anger **(techniques:** takeover management)
      pain **(techniques:** take over management, meaning questions)
      confusion **(techniques:** take over internal voices)

   3. postures **(techniques:** study in mindfulness)
   4. gestures **(techniques:** resist and study in mindfulness)
   5. tensions **(techniques:** study and go for meaning)
   6. images **(techniques:** gestalt or fantasy)

3. processing
   a. child **(techniques:** magical stranger)
   b. strong emotions **(techniques:** support spontaneous management behavior)
   c. going for meaning **(techniques:** meaning questions)

4. integration and completion **(techniques:** support spontaneous behavior and mind-body associations, probes, provide time and space to "cool down," homework, notice and contact completion)

Note: There are many ways to do Hakomi; this is an outline of my personal preferences. Other practitioners may do some of these things differently, without changing the basic nature of the method.

Bibliography

Anderson, Walt, *Open Secrets: A Western Guide to Tibetan Buddhism.* New York: Penguin Books, 1980.

Bandler, Richard and Grinder, John, *Structure of Magic,* Vol. 1. Palo Alto: Science and Behavior Books, Inc., 1975.

Becker, Robert O., M.D., and Selden, Gary, *The Body Electric.* New York: Quill Publications, of William Morrow, 1985.

Bradley, David, *Robert Frost: A Tribute to the Source.* New York: Holt, Rinehart and Winston: 1979.

Briggs, John and Peat, F. David, *Turbulent Mirror.* New York, Harper & Row, 1989.

Buber, Martin, *I and Thou.* New York: Collier Books, of MacMillan Publishing Company, 1958.

Capra Fritjof, *The Turning Point: Science and the Rising Culture.* Boston: Beacon Press, Inc., 1982.

Clark, Edward T., "Believing is Seeing- Not the Reverse". *the Quest,* Autumn, 1988 1.

Dyson, Freeman J., *Infinite In All Directions.* New York: Harper & Row, 1988.

Erickson, Milton H. and Rossi, Ernest and Sheila, *Hypnotic Realities.* New York: Irvington Publishers, Inc., 1976.

Feuerstein, Georg, *Structures of Consciousness.* Lower Lake, California, Integral Publishing, 1987

Gould, Stephen Jay, *Ever Since Darwin: reflections on natural history.* New York: Norton, c. 1977

Grossinger, Richard, *Planet Medicine.* Berkeley: North Atlantic Books, 1985.

Hofstadter, Douglas R., *Godel, Escher, Bach: An Eternal Golden Braid.* New York: Vintage Books, of Random House, 1980.

Jaynes, Julian, *The Origin of Consciousness in the Breakdown of the Bicameral Mind.* Boston: Houghton-Mifflin Co., 1977.

Johnson, Stephen, *Characterological Transformation.* New York: W.W. Norton, 1985.

Kurtz, Ron and Prestera, Hector, M.D., *The Body Reveals.* New York: Harper & Row, Publishers, 1976.

Lowen, Alexander, *Bioenergetics.* New York: Penguin Books, Inc., 1976.

Maturana, Humberto R. and Varela, Francisco J., *The Tree of Knowledge.* Boston: New Science Library, of Shambhala Publications, Inc., 1987.

Miller, James Grier, *Living Systems.* New York: McGraw-Hill Book Co., 1977.

Nhat Hanh, Thich, *The Miracle of Mindfulness!*. Boston: Beacon Press, 1976.

Pearson, Carol, *The Hero Within*. San Francisco: Harper & Row, Publishers, 1986.

Perls, Fritz, *Gestalt Therapy Verbatim*. Moab, UT, Real People Press, 1967.

Perls, Fritz and Hefferline, Ralph and Goodman, Paul, *Gestalt Therapy*. New York, Bantam Books, Inc., 1977.

Peterfreund, Emanuel, *The Process of Psychoanalytic Therapy*. Hillsdale, New Jersey, The Analytic Press, 1983

Rajneesh, Bhagwan Shree, *When the Shoe Fits*. India: Ma Yoga Laxmi Rajneesh Foundation,1976.

Rama, Swami and Ajaya, Swami, *Creative Use of Emotion*. Pennsylvania: Himalayan Internation Institute of Yoga Science and Philosophy of the U.S.A., 1976.

Reich, Wilhelm, *Character Analysis*. New York: Touchstone Books, Simon & Schuster, Inc., 1974.

Rinpoche, Kalu, *The Dharma That Illuminates All Beings Impartially Like the Light of the Sun and the Moon*. Albany, NY: State University of New York Press, 1986.

Rogers, Carl, *Client-Centered Therapy*. Boston: Houghton Miffin Co., 1951.

Rossi, Ernest Lawrence, *The Psychobiology of Mind-Body Healing*. New York: W. W. Norton & Company, 1986.

Schuurman, C.J., *Intrance*. Claremont, CA: Hunter House, Inc., 1984.

Shapiro, David, *Neurotic Styles*. New York: Basic Books, Inc., 1965.

Snyder, Gary, "Good, Wild, Sacred". In Jackson, Wes and Berry, Wendell, and Colman, Bruce (eds.), *Meeting the Expectations of the Land*. San Francisco: North Point Press, 1984.

Tart, Charles, *Waking Up*. Boston: New Science Library, of Shambhala Publications, Inc.: 1986.

Trungpa, Chogyam, "Becoming a Full Human Being" in Welwood, John, ed., *Awakening the Heart*. Boulder: Shambhala Publications, Inc., 1983.

von Bertalanffy, Ludwig, *A Systems View of Man*. Boulder, CO: Westview Press, Inc.,1981.

Watts, Alan and Chang-Liang, Al, *Tao: The Watercourse Way*. New York: Pantheon Books., Inc.

Webster's II New Riverside Dictionary, Boston: Houghton Mifflin, 1984.

Whitaker, Carl A. and Malone, Thomas P., *The Roots of Psychotherapy*. New York, Brunner/Mazel, 1981.

Wilber, Ken, *Eye To Eye*. Garden City, New York: Anchor Books, of Anchor Press/Doubleday, 1983.

Index

Contact:

Ron Kurtz Trainings, Inc.
P.O. Box 961
Ashland OR 97520

Email: ron@ronkurtz.com
Website: www.ronkurtz.com

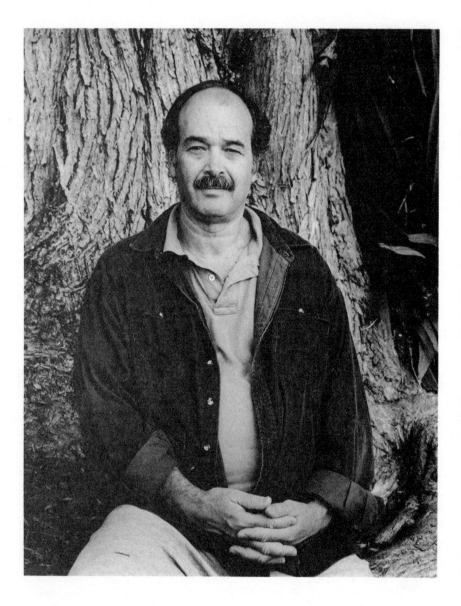

BIOGRAPHY

Ron Kurtz, a gifted therapist, writer, and teacher, developed the Hakomi Method in the mid 1970s as the culmination of his previous study and experience in psychology, science and philosophy. Influenced by the techniques of body-centered therapies (Bioenergetics, Gestalt, Feldenkrais and Structural Integration), by the intellectual breakthroughs of modern systems theory, and by the timeless spiritual principles of the East (particularly Taoism and Buddhism), Kurtz has created a synthesis that has special relevance for our time. He is the co-author of *The Body Reveals*. He did his undergraduate work in English and Physics and graduate work in Psychology. He is the founder and Director of the Hakomi Institute with offices in the United States, Canada and Europe.

LIFERHYTHM PUBLICATIONS

John C. Pierrakos M.D   CORE ENERGETICS
Developing the Capacity to Love and Heal
With 16 pages of four-color illustrations of human auras corresponding to their character structure,
300 pages
John C. Pierrakos, M.D., was a psychiatrist, body-therapist and an authority on consciousness and human energy fields. The focus of his work was to open the "Core" of his patients to a new awareness of how body, emotions, mind , will and spirituality form a unit. Dr. Pierrakos is considered one of the founders of a whole new movement in therapeutic work, integrating body, mind and spirit and this book has become classic.

John C. Pierrakos M.D.   EROS, LOVE & SEXUALITY
The Unifying Forces of Life and Relationship
122 pages
The free flow of the three great forces of life—eros, love and sexuality—is our greatest source of pleasure. These three forces are simply different aspects of the life force, and when we stay open, they are experienced as one. They generate all activity, all creativity.   John Pierrakos, the great psychiatrist, was a student and colleague of Wilhelm Reich, and co-founder of Bioenergetics; he later developed his own therapeutic work, Core Energetics, which integrates the higher dimensions into our physical existence.

Malcolm Brown, Ph.D.   THE HEALING TOUCH
An Introduction to Organismic Psychotherapy
320 pages   38 illustrations
A moving and meticulous account of Malcolm Brown's journey from Rogerian-style verbal psycho-therapist to gifted body psychotherapist.   Dr. Brown developed his own art and science of body psy-chotherapy with the purpose of re-activating the natural mental/spiritual polarities of the embodied soul and transcendental psyche.   Using powerful case histories as examples, Brown describes in the-ory and practice the development of his work; the techniques to awaken the energy flow and its inte-gration with the main Being centers: Eros, Logos, the Spirtual Warrior and the Hara.

Anna Halprin   RETURNING TO HEALTH
Returning to Health Through Movement & Imagery
195 pages   illustrations
Anna Halprin offers the wisdom of her dynamic life experience in the roles of dancer, teacher and healer. This book offers a theoretical and practical approach to using dance as a healing modality for people challenging cancer and other life-threatening illnesses.   In a clear and uplifting text, Anna Halprin, herself a cancer survivor, describes the expressive dance work she does with ill people. The book doc-uments a ten-week series with each class clearly described so that it can be easily used by other people interested in using dance as a healing art.

Bodo Baginski & Shalila Sharamon **REIKI** Universal Life Energy

200 pages illustrations

Reiki is described as the energy which forms the basis of all life. With the help of specific methods, anyone can learn to awaken and activate this universal life energy so that healing and harmonizing energy flows through the hands. Reiki is healing energy in the truest sense of the word, leading to greater individual harmony and attunement to the basic forces of the universe. This book features a unique compilation and interpretation, from the author's experience, of over 200 psychosomatic symptoms and diseases

Müller&Günther A COMPLETE BOOK OF
REIKI HEALING

Heal Yourself, Others, and the World Around You

192 pages, 85 photographs and illustrations

This book includes the history and practice of Reiki, with photographs and drawings as well as clear instructions for placement of hands in giving Reiki. Brigitte Müller was the first Reiki Master in Europe and she writes about her opening into a new world of healing with the freshness of discovery. Horst Günther experienced Reiki at one of Brigitte's first workshops in Germany, and it changed the course of his life. They share a vision of Reiki and the use of universal life energy to help us all heal ourselves and our world.

Fran Brown **LIVING REIKI: TAKATA'S TEACHINGS**

Stories from the Life of Hawayo Takata

110 pages

In this loving memoir to her teacher, Fran Brown has gathered the colorful stories told by Hawayo Takata during her thirty-five years s the only Reiki Master Teaching. The stories create an inspirational panorama of Takata's teachings, filled with the practical and spiritual aspects of a life given to healing.

Helmut G. Sieczka **CHAKRA BREATHING**

A Pathway to Energy and Harmony

100 pages Illustrations   *Supplemental Cassette Tape of Guided Meditations*

A guide to self-healing, this book is meant to help activate and harmonize the energy centers of the subtle body. The breath is the bridge between body and soul. In today's world as our lives are determined by stressful careers and peak performance, the silent and meditative moments have become more vital. Remembering our true selves, our natural energy balances are restored. Chakra-breathing enhances this kind of awareness and transformational work, especially on the emotional and energetic level.

R. Stamboliev **THE ENERGETICS OF
VOICE DIALOGUE**

Exploring the Energetics of Transformational Psychology

100 pages

Voice Dialogue is a therapeutic technique based on the transformational model of consciousness. This book approaches the human psyche as a synthesis of experience-patterns which may be modified only when the original pattern of an experience has been touched, understood and felt from an adult, integrated perspective, developing an "Aware Ego". This book explores the energetic aspects of the relationship between client and therapist, offering exercises for developing energetic skills and giving case histories to illustrate these skills. Voice Dialogue is the work of Hal and Sidra Stone Ph.Ds.

Allan Sachs D.C. The Authoritative Guide to
GRAPEFRUIT SEED EXTRACT
A Breakthrough in Alternative Treatment for Colds, Infections, Candida, Allergies, Herpes, Parasites & Many Other Ailments

Dr. Allan Sachs' revolutionary work in treating Candida albicans imbalance, food allergies and environmental illness has inspired thousands of patients and a generation of like-minded physicians. Based on his training as a medical researcher and his lifelong interest in plants, he undertook an intense study of the antimicrobial aspects of certain plant derivatives, expecially grapefruit seeds This is a complete handbook, giving information on the therapeutic use of grapefruit seed extract and its use for many household, farming, and industrial needs as well as for treating animals.

R. Flatischler **THE FORGOTTEN POWER OF RHYTHM**
TA KE TI NA

160 pages, illustrations

Rhythm is the central power of our lives; it connects us all. There is a powerful source of rhythmic knowledge in every human being. Reinhard Flatischler presents his brilliant approach to rhythm in this book, for both the layman and the professional musician. TA KE TI NA offers an experience of the interaction of pulse, breath, voice, walking and clapping which awakens our inherent rhythm in the most direct way—through the body. It provides a new understanding of the many musical voices of our world. *A companion CD of musical examples is available separately.*

Cousto **THE COSMIC OCTAVE**
Origin of Harmony

128 pages, 45 illustrations, numerous tables

Cousto demonstrates the direct relationship of astronomical data, such as the frequency of planetary orbits, to ancient and modern measuring systems, the human body, music and medicine. This book is compelling reading for all who wonder if a universal law of harmony does exist behind the apparent chaos of life. Tuning forks, tuned to the planets, earth, sun and moon, according to Cousto's calculations, are also available from LifeRhythm.

LifeRhythm

Books for Life Changes
P.O. Box 806   Mendocino CA 95460   USA
Tel: (707) 937-1825   Fax: (707) 937-3052
http://www.LifeRhythm.com
email: books@LifeRhythm.com